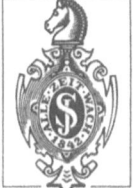

Subpulmonic Ventricular Septal Defect

Proceedings of the Third Asian Congress
of Pediatric Cardiology

Edited by
Hung-Chi Lue and Atsuyoshi Takao

With Contributions by
M. Ando, A.E. Becker, C.Y. Hong, C.R. Hung,
W.L. Lopez, H.C. Lue, I.P. Sukumar, A. Takao,
L.G. Van der Hauwaert, L.H.S. Van Mierop,
C. Vongprateep

Springer Japan KK

The Third Asian Congress of Pediatric Cardiology held in Taipei, November 1983

Hung-Chi Lue
Professor and Chairman
Department of Pediatrics
College of Medicine
National Taiwan University
Taipei, Taiwan, R.O.C.

Atsuyoshi Takao
Professor of
Pediatric Cardiology
Director of
The Heart Institute of Japan
Tokyo Women's Medical College
Tokyo, Japan

Library of Congress Cataloging-in-Publication Data

Asian Congress of Pediatric Cardiology (3rd: 1983#: Taipei, Taiwan)
Subpulmonic ventricular septal defect.
Conference held in Taipei on Nov. 28, 1983.
Includes bibliographies and index.
1. Ventricular septal defects — Congresses.
2. Aortic value — Abnormalities — Congresses.
3. Ventricular septal defects — Asia — Congresses.
4. Aortic valve — Abnormalities — Asia — Congresses.
I. Lue, Hung-Chi, 1931-   II. Takao, Atsuyoshi.
III. Ando, M. (Masahiko) IV. Title. [DNLM: 1. Aortic Valve — abnormalities — congresses. 2. Heart Septal Defects, Ventricular — congresses. W3 AS144P 3rd 1983s/WG 220 A832 1983s]
RJ426.V4A75 1983   616.1'2   86-17719

ISBN 978-4-431-70014-2   ISBN 978-4-431-68375-9 (eBook)
DOI 10.1007/978-4-431-68375-9

© Springer Japan 1986
Originally published by Springer-Verlag Tokyo in 1986.

Typesetting: Koford Prints (Pte.) Ltd., Singapore

Preface

The Asian Society of Pediatric Cardiology has advocated the importance, since its founding in 1976, of studying and disseminating knowledge about the important cardiovascular diseases prevalent in Asia. Subpulmonic ventricular septal defect, reportedly more common among Japanese than among Occidentals, swiftly became a focus of attention. Soon after the Second Asian Congress of Pediatric Cardiology, held at Bangkok in 1979, fellow Asian pediatric cardiologists resolved to study this problem, and the main theme of the next Congress was scheduled to be "Is Subpulmonic Ventricular Septal Defect an Oriental Disease?". Prospective as well as retrospective studies were encouraged, the results to be presented and discussed at the Congress. The Third Asian Congress of Pediatric Cardiology was held in Taipei on November 28, 1983. Distinguished pathologists, cardiologists, and surgeons from the US, UK, Belgium, and the Netherlands — Drs. L.H.S. Van Mierop, S. Blumenthal, D. McNamara, J. Malm, N. Talner, J. Somerveille, J. Stark, L.G. Van der Hauwaert, and A.E. Becker — were invited to present their work and actively participate in the Congress. The important data thus gathered from both Asian and Western countries, and some results of the lively debates enjoyed during the Congress, are included in this volume.

The expert views on the development of the ventricular septum and the classification of ventricular septal defects appearing in this volume are most succinct and informative. The discussions of the nomenclature of each subtype of ventricular septal defect are comprehensive. The pathologic anatomy of the ventricular septal defect with aortic valve prolapse and regurgitation, and the related developmental mechanisms, are masterfully depicted, based on extensive and thorough studies. The state of the art in research on ventricular septal defect and coronary cusp prolapse is reported from Belgium, India, Indonesia, Japan, Korea, the Philippines, and Taiwan, allowing us to compare the incidence of ventricular septal defect with cusp prolapse and to perceive the extent of the problem it causes in the respective countries.

Spontaneous closure of the defect occurs in 30% to 50% or more of the patients with subaortic or so-called perimembranous ventricular septal defect. Closure rarely occurs, however, in those with subpulmonic ventricular septal defect, which predisposes to development of coronary cusp prolapse with or without aortic regurgitation. Surgical repair of the subpulmonic ventricular septal defect helps prevent further prolapsing of the coronary cusp. The natural history of this important disease, prevalent among Orientals, has thus become better understood.

The argument over "Who are Orientals?" continues; however, the definition can best be made on the basis of various genetic traits and anthropological features.

Acknowledgements. We would like to thank Drs. Laura C.C. Meng, Wen-Jen Su and the other members of the Organizing Committee for the Third Asian Congress of Pediatric Cardiology. Without their planning and hard work, such a successful Congress would not have been possible. We would like to acknowledge the invaluable advice of Drs. Sanji Kuaskawa and Choompol Vongprateep, former presidents of the Asian Society of Pediatric Cardiology. We are grateful to the members of the Editorial Board of "Heart and Vessels," and also to those of the staff of Springer-Verlag Tokyo who have provided valuable advice and guidance. The holding of the Congress and the publication of this book were made possible by grants from the National Science Council, Republic of China, and the Heart Institute of Japan.

Hung-Chi Lue and Atsuyoshi Takao

Table of Contents

Treatment of ventricular septal defect and coronary cusp prolapse

Contributors and Participants

Masahiko Ando, M.D.
Associate Professor of Pediatric Cardiology, The Heart Institute of Japan, Tokyo Women's Medical College, Tokyo, Japan

Anton E. Becker, M.D.
Professor of Pathology, Academic Medical Center, University of Amsterdam, The Netherlands

Sidney Blumenthal, M.D.
Special Consultant to Vice President for Health Sciences, Columbia University, New York, N.Y., U.S.A.; Formerly: Director, Division of Heart and Vascular Diseases, National Heart and Lung Institute, Bethesda, Maryland, U.S.A.

Shu-Hsun Chu, M.D.
Professor of Surgery, Department of Surgery, National Taiwan University College of Medicine, Taipei, Taiwan, R.O.C.

Asikin Hanafiah, M.D.
Professor of Pediatrics, Department of Pediatrics, University of Indonesia, Jakarta, Indonesia

Chang-Yee Hong, M.D.
Professor of Pediatrics, Department of Pediatrics, Seoul National University, Seoul, Korea

Chi-Ren Hung, M.D.
Professor of Surgery, Department of Surgery, National Taiwan University College of Medicine, Taipei, Taiwan, R.O.C.

Wilberto L. Lopez, M.D.
Head, Department of Pediatric Cardiology, Philippine Heart Center for Asia, Manila, The Philippines

Hung-Chi Lue, M.D.
Professor and Chairman, Department of Pediatrics, National Taiwan University College of Medicine, Taipei, Taiwan, R.O.C.

James R. Malm, M.D.
Professor of Surgery, College of Physicians and Surgeons, Columbia University, New York, N.Y., U.S.A.

Dan G. McNamara, M.D.
Chief of Pediatric Cardiology and Professor of Medicine, Section of Cardiology, Department of Pediatrics, Baylor College of Medicine and Texas Children's Hospital, Houston, Texas, U.S.A.

C.C. Laura Meng, M.D.
Professor of Pediatrics, Department of Pediatrics, Veterans General Hospital, Taipei, Taiwan, R.O.C.

Masahiko Okuni, M.D.
Professor and Chairman, Department of Pediatrics, Nihon University School of Medicine, Tokyo, Japan

Lily I. Rilantono, M.D.
Professor of Pediatrics, Department of Pediatrics, University of Indonesia, Jakarta, Indonesia

Jane Somerville, M.D.
Pediatric and Adolescent Unit, National Heart Hospital, London, U.K.

Jaroslav Stark, M.D.
Cardiothoracic Surgeon, The Hospital for Sick Children, London, U.K.

I.P. Sukumar, M.D.
Professor and Head, Cardiology Department, Christian Medical College and Hospital, Vellore, India

Atsuyoshi Takao, M.D.
Professor of Pediatric Cardiology, Director, The Heart Institute of Japan, Tokyo Women's Medical College, Tokyo, Japan

Norman S. Talner, M.D.
Professor of Pediatrics, Department of Pediatrics, Yale University Medical Center, New Haven, Connecticut, U.S.A.

Katsuhiko Tatsuno, M.D.
Chief Surgeon, Sakakibara Heart Institute, Tokyo, Japan

L.G. Van der Hauwaert, M.D.
Professor of Pediatrics, Department of Pediatric Cardiology, University Hospital Gasthuisberg, Leuven, Belgium

L.H.S. Van Mierop, M.D.
Graduate Research Professor, Department of Pediatrics, Division of Cardiology and Research, University of Florida College of Medicine, Gainesville, Florida, U.S.A.

Choompol Vongprateep, M.D.
Chief, Pediatric Cardiology Service, Children's Hospital, Bangkok, Thailand

Introduction

Is subpulmonic ventricular septal defect an Oriental disease?

Hung-Chi Lue

Ventricular septal defect (VSD) is the most common congenital cardiac malformation, occurring as an isolated or prime lesion in 20%-30% of all infants and children with congenital heart disease in Western countries [1-3] as well as in Japan [4]. A study of 3891 Chinese infants and children with congenital heart disease also showed a similar frequency of 31.2% (Table 1). VSD occurs as a result of deficiency of ventricular substance or of fusion failure between each of the four developmental components of the ventricular septum, namely: (1) the conus or muscular outlet septum; (2) membranous septum; (3) sinus or muscular inlet septum; and (4) muscular trabecular septum (Fig. 1) [5]. To identify clinically and specifically conus, membranous, sinus, or trabecular septal defects is usually difficult, except in patients whose cardiac murmur is characteristically blowing and pansystolic, best heard in the second and third left interspaces, allowing clinicians to label it as conus septal defect or so-called subpulmonic VSD [6-8]. Since the introduction of powerful biplane cineangiocardiography and more recently of 2-D echocardiography, precise identification of the type of VSD has become not only clinically possible but also necessary, particularly so when corrective surgery is contemplated [6-11].

Classification and terminology of VSDs

To date, the classifications and terminologies of VSDs appearing in the literature have been innumerable and have varied widely, leading often to ambiguity or even confusion, making VSDs hard to understand. In 1957, Kirklin and his associates [12] classified VSDs into four general types according to anatomic location at surgery: Type I, the defect beneath the pulmonary valve and above the crista supraventricularis; type II, the defect inferior to the crista supraventracularis and immediately beneath the aortic valve, involving the membranous septum; type III, the defect related to the inflow tract and beneath the septal leaflet of the tricuspid valve; type IV, near the apex of the muscular septum. In 1962, Cooley and co-workers [13] similarly classified the VSDs of their surgical patients into four types. Based on development aspects, Goor and associates [5] in 1970 classified VSDs into as many as 13 specific types, namely infundibular types I-V, membranous, atrioventricular septal defect, sinus (or smooth) types I-V, and trabeculated. In 1980, Soto and associates [14] considered the ventricular septum as possessing either a membranous or muscular portion, and they termed the defect involving the

Address reprint request to: Hung-Chi Lue, M.D., No.1, Chang-teh St., National Taiwan University Hospital, Taipei, Taiwan, R.O.C. 100

membranous septum perimembranous VSD; this was because they found that it was found invariably to have additional involvement of the surrounding muscular septum extending into either the inlet, trabecular, or outlet (infundibular) septum [14]. They termed the defect within the three muscular septa muscular outlet, muscular inlet, and muscular trabecular, respectively [14]. They specifically called the defect in the upper-most area of the conus or muscular outlet septum, subjacent to both pulmonary and

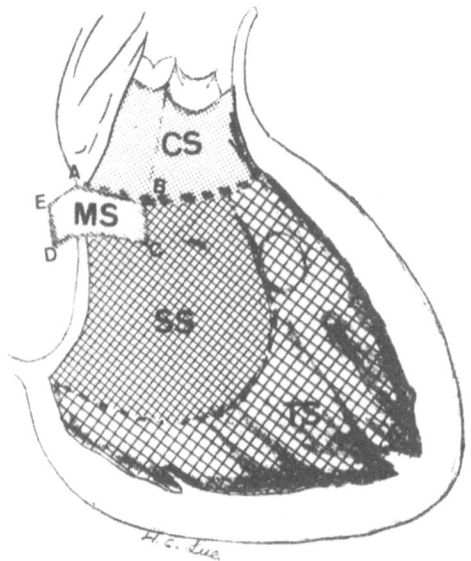

Fig. 1. Four developmental components of the ventricular septum, viewed from right ventricle. *CS* conus septum, *MS, ABCDE* membranous septum, *SS* sinus septum, *TS* trabecular septum. Modified from Goor et al. [5]

Table 1. Frequency of occurrence of major cardiac malformations

Disease	Percentage
Ventricular septal defect	31.2
Tetralogy of Fallot	22.0
Patent ductus arteriosus	11.8
Pulmonary stenosis	6.3
Transposition of great arteries	5.5
Atrial septal defect	4.9
Dextrocardia	2.1
Coarctation of aorta	1.7
Endocardial cushion defect	1.6
Double-outlet right ventricle	1.3
Anomalous pulmonary venous return	1.3
Persistent truncus arteriosus	1.1
Aortic stenosis	0.9
Tricuspid atresia	0.8
All others	5.9

Data based on 3891 infants and children with congenital heart disease, classified according to one major diagnosis made by catheterization, surgery, and/or autopsy, National Taiwan University Hospital, September 1960 to June 1985

aortic valves, a subarterial outlet defect [14]. The perimembranous VSD differs from the muscular defect in that the former always has a remnant of the membranous septum and a direct relationship with the atrioventricular conduction bundle [14, 15].

A modified classification of VSDs for clinical application

For purposes of clinical application, a modified classification of VSDs is suggested and many of the analogies or synonyms are grouped accordingly (Table 2).

I. Subpulmonic VSD: Included in this general type are the defects located in the uppermost, mid, or entire portion of the conus or muscular outlet septum, without involvement of the membranous septum [6, 11, 12, 16–20].

II. Subaortic VSD: Pertaining to this general type are by far the most common ventricular septal defects occurring in the area of the membranous septum, including those extending into part of the outlet, inlet, or trabecular septum [14, 16, 18]. Included in this category is also the defect in the atrioventricular part of the membranous septum (above the tricuspid annulus), called atrioventricular septal defect [3, 5, 32].

III. Atrioventricular (AV) canal VSD: Included here is the defect involving both membranous and inlet or so-called sinus septa with stigmata of the atrioventricular canal [19, 31, 35]. ECG shows almost invariably a superior axis deviation of the mean electrical axis of the QRS complex. The atrioventricular valve may be involved, leaving a cleft [31].

IV. Muscular VSD: Included in this general type are the defects occurring in the muscular inlet septum or trabecular septum. The muscular inlet VSD is completely

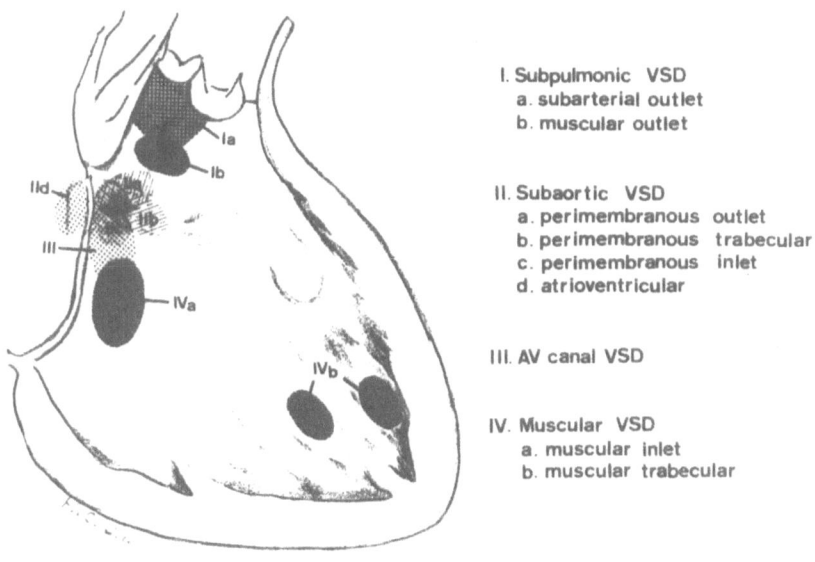

I. Subpulmonic VSD
   a. subarterial outlet
   b. muscular outlet

II. Subaortic VSD
    a. perimembranous outlet
    b. perimembranous trabecular
    c. perimembranous inlet
    d. atrioventricular

III. AV canal VSD

IV. Muscular VSD
    a. muscular inlet
    b. muscular trabecular

Fig. 2. General and specific types of ventricular septal defects and their classification. Modified from Goor et al. [5] and Soto et al. [14]

Table 2. A modified classification of ventricular septal defects and grouping of terminologies appearing in the literature

Type of VSD (developmental components involved)	Synonyms and analogies
I. Subpulmonic VSD [6, 11, 16–20] (conus septum, in general)	Type I [12, 13], conus [7, 21, 22] infundibular [5, 32], bulbar [23, 24], supracristal [5, 6, 11, 17, 24–26], high [28, 29]
a. Subarterial outlet [14] (distal portion of conus septum)	Subarterial infundibular [14], distal conus [27, 32], infundibular type III [5]
b. Muscular outlet [14] (midportion of conus septum)	Muscular infundibular [14], midconus [5, 32], midcristal [5], infundibular type II [5]
c. Total outlet (entire conus septum)	Total conus [32], absent cristal [5], infundibular type IV [5]
II. Subaortic VSD [16, 18] (membranous septum, in general)	Type II [12, 13], membranous [2, 5, 22, 25, 32,], subcristal [20], infracristal [17, 24, 26], low [29], high [30], outflow [3]
III. AV canal VSD [19, 31, 35] (membranous and sinus septa)	Endocardial cushion defect type [12, 31], type III [12, 13], canal [32], smooth type II [5], persistent common atrioventricular canal type [31], posterior (confluent type) [10, 35] perimembranous inlet with gross deficiency of inlet septum [14]
IV. Muscular VSD [32] a. Muscular inlet [14] (sinus septum)	Type III [12, 13], posterior (muscular) [10], muscular posterior [14], inflow [3], smooth type III, IV, IV [5], smooth [32]
b. Muscular trabecular [5, 14] (trabecular septum)	Type IV [12, 13], trabeculated [5, 14], muscular [17], low [12], apical [32], Swiss cheese type [30]

surrounded by muscle without involving the membranous septum. This defect has often been included in AV canal VSD or so-called type III VSD [12, 13]. Left ventricular angiocardiograms usually show no stigmata of the atrioventricular canal, and ECG reveals no superior axis deviation of the QRS axis. Separation of this muscular inlet VSD from muscular trabecular defect is possible clinically only by 2-D echocardiography or selective left ventriculography, especially axial cineangiography [9, 10]. The muscular trabecular VSD may be single or multiple [12–14, 32].

Special features of subpulmonic VSD

Sakakibara [27] and Tatsuno and co-workers [7] reported a higher incidence of subpulmonic VSD among Japanese than among Occidentals. The percentage incidence of subpulmonic VSD among all VSDs in Japan was approximately 30%, while that in the USA and Western European countries was only 6%–8% (Table 3) [6, 7, 13, 25]. In Taiwan, the rate was also high, 36.8% among surgical cases of all ages [36] and 22.6% among infants and children of VSD prospectively studied (unpublished observation). The incidence of subpulmonic VSD in other Oriental countries remains to be found. While more than half of the VSDs spontaneously closed [1, 4], very rarely did the subpulmonic VSD. An important complication — prolapse of the aortic valve and sinus of Valsalva with or without aortic regurgitation — occurs more frequently in patients with subpulmonic than in those with subaortic VSD [27]. More accurate figures on the incidence of this complication remain to be studied. The indications for and timing of surgery in patients with such a complication are still matters of conjecture and argument, posing interesting but difficult problems for pediatric cardiologists and cardiac surgeons [33, 34]. The development of the conal septum in Orientals appears to differ from that in Occidentals. "Is subpulmonic ventricular septal defect an Oriental disease?" It is timely and relevant that this important question be discussed and answered by fellow Asian pediatric cardiologists together with distinguished physicians, surgeons, and investigators from all over the world at the Third Asian Congress of Pediatric Cardiology held in Taipei on December 1, 1983.

Table 3. A comparison of the anatomic position of ventricular septal defects in various countries

Type of VSD	USA Becu et al. [25] ($n=50$)[a]	USA Cooley et al. [13] ($n=300$)[b]	US, UK, Holland Soto et al. [14] ($n=220$)[a]	Japan Ando et al. [32] ($n=146$)[a]	Japan Tatsuno [7] ($n=551$)[b]	Taiwan Chu et al. [36] ($n=315$)[b]	Taiwan Lue et al. ($n=332$)[c]
Subpulmonic[d]	8	5.7	6.9	30.9	31.6	36.8	22.6
Subaortic	70	79.3	69.6	52	66.1	61.3	75.0
AV canal type	8	3.7	6.8	1.4	1.8	1.6	0.9
Muscular	12	3.0	18.2	15.7	0.5	0.3	0.6
Others	2	8.3	1.4	—	—	—	0.9

[a] Autopsy series [b] Surgical series of all ages [c] Pediatric series prospectively studied [d] Including midconus and subarterial outlet VSDs

References

1. Hoffman JIE (1968) Natural history of congenital heart disease. Problems in its assessment with special reference to ventricular septal defect. Circulation 37: 97–125
2. Keith JD, Rowe RD, Vlad P (1978) Heart disease in infancy and childhood (3rd edn). Macmillan, New York, pp 320–321
3. Edwards JE (1960) Congenital malformations of the heart and great vessels. In: Gould SE (ed) Pathology of the heart, Thomas, Springfield, Ill.
4. Yokoyama M, Takao A, Sakakibara S (1970) Natural history and surgical indications of ventricular septal defect. Am Heart J 80: 597–605
5. Goor DA, Lillehei CW, Rees R, Edwards JE (1970) Isolated ventricular septal defect. Developmental basis for various types and presentation of classification. Chest 58: 468–482
6. Steinfeld L, Dimich I, Park SC, Baron MG (1972) Clinical diagnosis of isolated subpulmonic (supra-, cristal) ventricular septal defect. Am J Cardiol 30: 19–24
7. Tatsuno K, Ando M, Takao A, Hatsune K, Konno S (1975) Diagnostic importance of aortography in conal ventricular septal defect. Am Heart J 89: 171–177
8. Farru O, Duffau G, Rodriguez R (1971) Auscultatory and phono-cardiographic characteristics of supracristal ventricular septal defect. Br Heart J 33: 238–245
9. Bargeron LM Jr, Elliot LP, Soto B, Bream PR, Curry GC (1977) Axial cineangiography in congenital heart disease. Section I. Concept, technical and anatomical considerations. Circulation 56: 1075–83

10. Green CE, Elliot LP, Bargeron LM Jr (1981) Axial cineangiographic evaluation of the posterior ventricular septal defect. Am J Cardiol 48: 331–335
11. Baron MG, Wolf BS, Steinfeld L (1968) Angiographic diagnosis of subpulmonic ventricular septal defect. Am J Roentgen 103: 93–103
12. Kirklin JW, Harshbarger HG, Donald DE, Edwards JE (1957) Surgical correction of ventricular septal defect: Anatomic and technical considerations. J Thorac Surg 33: 45–59
13. Cooley DA, Garrett HE, Howard HS (1962) The surgical treatment of ventricular septal defect: An analysis of 300 consecutive surgical cases. Prog Cardiovasc Dis 4: 312–323
14. Soto B, Becker AE, Moulaert AJ, Lie JT, Anderson RH (1980) Classification of ventricular septal defect. Br Heart J 43: 332–343
15. Milo S, Ho SY, Wilkinson JL, Anderson RH (1980) Surgical anatomy and atrioventricular conduction tissues of hearts with isolated ventricular septal defects. J Thorac Cardiovasc Surg 79: 244–255
16. Keane JF, Plauth WH, Nadas AS (1977) Ventricular septal defect with aortic regurgitation. Circulation (Suppl) 56: 72–77
17. Kozuka T, Nosaki T, Sato K (1970) Ventricular septal defect in tetralogy of Fallot. Am J Roentgenol Radium Ther Nucl Med 110: 497–504
18. Rao BNS, Edwards JE (1974) Conditions simulating the tetralogy of Fallot. Circulation 49: 173–178
19. Blackstone EH, Kirklin JW, Bradley EL, DuShane JW, Appelbaum A (1976) Optimal age and results in repair of large ventricular septal defects. J Thorac Cardiovasc Surg 72: 661–679
20. Van Praagh R, McNamara JJ (1968) Anatomic types of ventricular septal defect with aortic insufficiency: Diagnostic and surgical considerations. Am Heart J 75: 604–619
21. Ando M (1974) Subpulmonic ventricular septal defect with pulmonary stenosis. Circulation 50: 412
22. Selzer A (1949) Defects of the ventricular septum. Summary of twelve cases and review of the literature. Arch Intern Med 84: 798
23. Abbott ME (1936) Atlas of congenital cardiac disease. Am Heart Assoc, New York
24. Somerville J, Brandao A, Ross DN (1970) Aortic regurgitation with ventricular septal defect. Surgical management and clinical features. Circulation 41: 317–330
25. Becu LM, Fontana RS, DuShane JW, Kirklin JW, Burchell HB, Edwards JE (1956) Anatomic and pathologic studies in ventricular septal defect. Circulation 14: 349–364
26. Jaffe RB, Scherer JL (1977) Supracristal ventricular septal defects: Spectrum of associated lesions and complications. Am J Roentgenol 128: 629–637
27. Sakakibara S (1974) Experiences with congenital anomalies of the heart in Japan. J Thorac Cardiovasc Surg 68: 190–195
28. Lev M (1959) The pathologic anatomy of ventricular septal defect. Dis Chest 35: 533–545
29. Nadas AS, Thilenius OG, LaFarge CG, Hauck AJ (1964) Ventricular septal defect with aortic regurgitation: Medical and pathologic aspects. Circulation 29: 862–873
30. Kirklin JW, McGoon DC, DuShane JW (1960) Surgical treatment of ventricular septal defect. J Thorac Cardiovasc Surg 40: 763–775
31. Neufeld HN, Titus JD, DuShane JW, Burchell HB, Edwards JE (1961) Isolated ventricular septal defect of the persistent common atrio-ventricular canal type. Circulation 23: 685–697
32. Ando M, Takao A, Mori K (1977) In: Inoue E, Nishimura H (eds) Genetic and environmental factors in congenital heart disease: Genetic environmental interaction in common disease. University of Tokyo Press, Tokyo, pp 71–87
33. Blumenthal S, Malm JR, Ellis K (1967) Natural history of ventricular septal defect with aortic valve prolapse (Abstract). Circulation 35, 36: 11–73
34. Tatsuno K, Konno S, Ando M, Sakakibara S (1973) Pathogenetic mechanisms of prolapsing aortic valve and aortic regurgitation associated with ventricular septal defect. Anatomical, angiographic, and surgical considerations. Circulation 48: 1028–1037
35. Kiely B, Adams P Jr, Anderson RC, Lester RG (1958) The ostium primum syndrome. AMA J Dis Child 96: 381–403
36. Chu SH, Hung CR, Yang YJ (1980) Surgical treatment of congenital ventricular septal defects. I. Anatomical classification of congenital ventricular septal defects in Chinese and its clinical implications. J Formosan Med Assoc 79: 1018–1024

Pathology and diagnosis of ventricular septal defect and coronary cusp prolapse

Development of the ventricular septum of the heart*

Lodewyk H.S. Van Mierop and Lynn M. Kutsche

In man, development of the cardiovascular system begins in embryos of about 3 weeks ovulation age and is essentially completed 3 weeks later. Cardiovascular development, therefore, takes place very early and proceeds rapidly. This is a major reason why the study of cardiovascular development is difficult. Events of major importance for the understanding of the processes which lead to cardiac septation and the formation of atrioventricular and arterial valves take place so quickly and are so elusive that we still don't have a thorough understanding of what exactly happens. These uncertainties continue to fuel controversies concerning not only normal cardiovascular development but also the pathogenesis of congenital cardiac defects. Considerable progress, however, has been made in the past few decades [1-9] and the blanks in our knowledge and understanding of heart development are becoming fewer and smaller.

Septum formation in the developing embryo

Partitions can be formed in the early embryonic heart in one of two ways depending upon the structure of the heart wall in the particular section to be divided [5] (Fig. 1):

1. If the wall of the segment of heart to be partitioned is thin and consists almost exclusively of myocardium, then rapid and expansive growth of this segment on either side of a narrow section which increases in diameter only slowly or not at all will produce an incomplete septum. The portions of the walls of the expanded regions on either side of the narrow intervening segment eventually appose and generally fuse. If expansive growth takes place in all directions, the particular portion of the heart after fusion of the apposing walls is transformed into a structure containing a diaphragm with a central opening. More often, however, expansive growth takes place mainly in one direction, resulting in formation of a septum with an excentrically placed communication between the two adjoining chambers. A septum formed in this fashion is simply a reduplication of the organ wall and is never complete. There is always an opening in the septum which has a diameter at least equal to that of the original lumen. If fusion of the apposing walls occurs early and keeps pace with the expansive growth of the cardiac section involved, it may never be very obvious that the septum is a reduplication and it may look more like a ridge (muscular ventricular septum) or a membrane (atrial septum primum).

* This paper appeared in Heart and Vessels Vol. 1, No. 1 (1985).

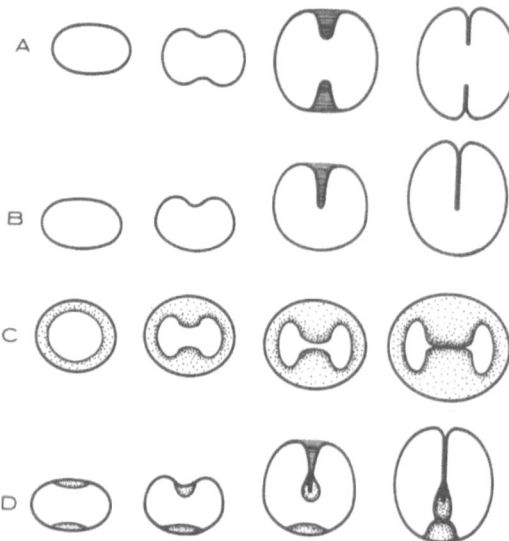

Fig. 1A-D. Mechanisms of cardiac septation. **A, B** passively formed septum. **C** actively formed septum. **D** combination of **B** and **C** (from [15])

2 In sections of the early embryonic heart which possess a well-developed layer of cardiac mesenchyme (endocardial cushion tissue) between the myocardium and the endocardium, e.g. the atrioventricular canal, the conus cordis and the truncus arteriosus, septation takes place in a quite different fashion. Local elaborations of cardiac mesenchyme form two opposing masses of tissue which grow towards each other and fuse. Such masses of cardiac mesenchyme are always large and bulky and are commonly referred to as "cushions" or "swellings". When fully formed, septa developed in this fashion are complete and their thickness characteristically equals or exceeds their height in the early phases of development.

Once fusion of opposing endocardial cushions has occured there is little if any further growth of the mesenchymal, embryonic septum thus formed. This limited growth capacity of cushion tissue was already commented upon by Grant [10]. Endocardial cushion tissue eventually either disappears completely or is replaced by connective tissue. As the heart grows and the lumen on either side of the mesenchymal septum expands, the septum is enlarged essentially in the same manner as described above. The result, therefore, is a septum which consists of myocardium with a narrow central area consisting of endocardial cushion tissue. Since this tissue often disappears completely, the end result is a complete septum consisting of myocardium. The crista supraventricularis of the right ventricle is an example of a structure formed in this fashion. Occasionally, both in normal and congenitally defective hearts, the area of fusion is still visible. The older view that a muscular septum is formed to its full extent by cardiac mesenchyme which is then secondarily invaded by myocardium, is no longer tenable. That embryonic cardiac septa which consit of endocardial cushion tissue, e.g. the embryonic conal septum and the atrioventricular canal septum, contribute very little if any to either the formation of the cardiac septum or the atrioventricular valves has been recognized only recently. They do have to develop normally however, for a normal septum to become established. Their minimal contribution to the post natal septum has been shown recently by the elegant studies of De la Cruz et al. [9] who introduced markers in the endocardial cushions of the early embryonic heart and were able to trace their fate throughout development.

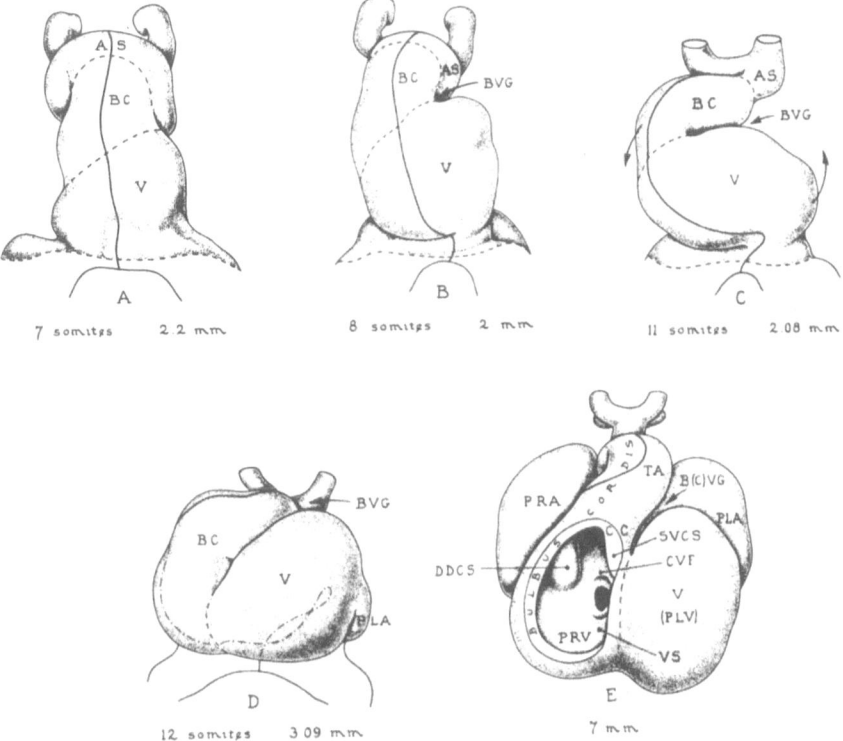

Fig. 2A-E. Formation of cardiac loop. Changing position of black line drawn on what was the ventral surface of the heart tube, **A**, shows the amount of torsion induced by cardiac looping. Note the elongation of the heart tube is mainly due to growth of the bulbus cordis, *BC* (**A** *AS* aortic sac, *V* ventricle. **B** *BVG* bulboventricular groove, *PRA* primitive right atrium, *PRV* primitive right ventricle, *VS* ventricular septum, *PLV* primitive left ventricle, *CVF* conoventricular flange, *SVCS* sinistroventral conus cushion, *B(C)VG* bulbo-(cono) ventricular groove, *TA* truncus arteriosus, *CC* conus cordis). Modified after Davis [11], from [1]

Formation of the heart loop

In a human embryo of about 7 somites (approximately 23 days ovulation age), the heart is essentially a straight tube, the bulboventricular tube, which lies within the pericardial cavity. With further growth the bulboventricular tube bends to the right and anteriorly, initially into the shape of the letter "C" and later into a compound sigmoid structure, the bulboventricular loop (Fig.2). The deepening concavity on the left side of the bulboventricular loop is referred to as the bulboventricular groove, which corresponds internally to the bulboventricular (later conoventricular) fold. The free border of the bulboventricular fold forms part of the circumference of the bulboventricular (later primary interventricular) foramen, a relatively narrow segment of the bulboventricular loop. Expansive growth on either side produces the embryonic ventricle on the left (proximally) and the bulbus cordis on the right (distally). The atrioventricular junction which at first lies in the midline, is crowded laterally and to the left.

After the heart loop has been formed diverticula appear along the ventrolateral borders

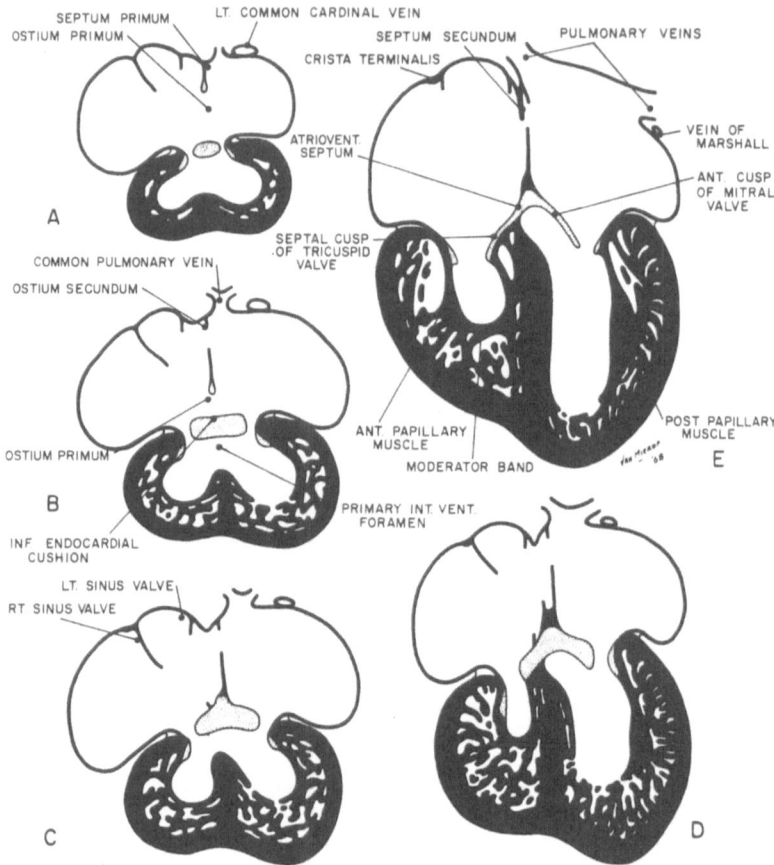

Fig. 3A-E. Sections through the heart of embryos. **A** 6-mm C-R length, stage XIV. **B** 9-mm, stage XVI. **C** 12-mm, stage XVII. **D** 17-mm, stage XVIII. **E** 40-mm, diagrammatic. (From Van Mierop LHS (1978) Embryology of the atrioventricular canal region and pathogeneses of endocardial cushion defects. In: Feldt RH (ed) Atrioventricular canal defects. Saunders, Philadelphia)

of the heart tube in the early embryonic ventricle and in the proximal part of the bulbus cordis on either side of the bulboventricular foramen. These diverticula initially develop at the expense of a thick layer of nearly acellular tissue (termed "cardiac jelly" by Davis [11]) which lines the interior of the bulboventricular loop. Later the diverticula become more numerous and penetrate the mycocardium as the latter increases in thickness. Thus the lumen of both the embryonic ventricle and bulbus cordis increase in capacity (Fig. 3).

The trabeculated embryonic ventricle may now be called the primitive left ventricle since it will contribute the major portion of the left ventricle. Similarly, the proximal 1/3 of the bulbus cordis, also trabeculated, may be called the primitive right ventricle. At this stage of development the embryo is approximately 3 mm long and has an ovulation age of about 25 days. Because of the formation of cardiac chambers and cardiac septa it becomes helpful to distinguish 3 sections in the bulbus cordis of which the proximal trabe-culated 1/3 is the primitive right ventricle. From the adjacent middle 1/3 of the bulbus, the conus cordis, the outflow portions of both ventricles will be derived. The terminal 1/3 after partitioning develops into the aortic and pulmonary roots and may therefore be referred to as the truncus arteriosus.

The rapid growth and expansion of the atria causes the truncoconal section of the bulbus cordis to shift from its initial far lateral position in a embryo of about 3 mm long to a more medial location as seen in an embryo of about 5 mm crown-rump (C-R) length. The truncus arteriosus comes to lie in a midsagittal position in a depression of the atrial roof. The conus cordis assumes an oblique position. At this stage of development the external shape of the heart already suggests its future four-chambered condition (Fig. 2). Internally, however, it still consists essentially of a single convoluted tube with a number of local expansions representing the primitive atria and ventricles. The still undivided atrioventricular canal connects the common atrium to the primitive left ventricle and blood can reach the primitive right ventricle only by way of the primary interventricular foramen, the inferior and anterior borders of which are formed by the developing muscular ventricular septum and the superior and posterior borders by the bulboventricular fold.

Development of the muscular ventricular septum

On either side of the primary ventricular foramen the ventricles enlarge by growth of the myocardial wall. This growth process, however, is always closely followed by increased diverticulation and formation of trabeculae which on the one hand increases the capacity of the ventricles and on the other prevents the myocardial wall becoming too thick and solid. The original free lumen of the ventricle retains its configuration for some time, which results in the heart for a time having a very small free lumen and a large mass of trabeculae enclosed by a rather thin outer layer of compact myocardium (Fig. 3). This gives the ventricles a spongy appearance, a condition which in many lower animals persists into the adult state [12], but in birds and mammals most of the trabeculae normally disappear once functional arterial valves have been formed.

The medial walls of the growing and expanding ventricles appose and fuse, creating the major portion of the muscular ventricular septum. On the right side a large trabecula, the trabecula septomarginalis, appears early in development and runs from the antero-inferior border of the primary interventricular foramen towards the apicolateral wall where it loses itself among parietal trabeculae. The primary interventricular foramen never closes but actually enlarges and in the fully developed heart it gives access to the aortic infundibulum or vestibule.

In embryos of about 6 mm C-R length the atrioventricular canal and the truncoconal region of the embryonic heart have shifted medially from the far lateral position seen in younger specimens. However, the atrioventricular canal still gives access only to the primitive left ventricle and is separated from the conus cordis by the cono-(bulbo) ventricular fold. The center portion of this fold effaces and blood can now enter the primitive right ventricle directly from the atrium. The right sided portion of the conoventricular fold persists to become part of the parietal band of the postnatal heart, the left extremity usually blends with the left ventricular wall, but may remain visible as the anterolateral muscle bundle [13]. Because of the shift to the left and eventual effacement of the central part of the fold, the plane of the primary interventricular foramen comes to incline more and more to the left from an originally vertical position. Thus, direct access is gained from the primitive left ventricle to the posteromedial portion of the conus cordis and from there to the aorta.

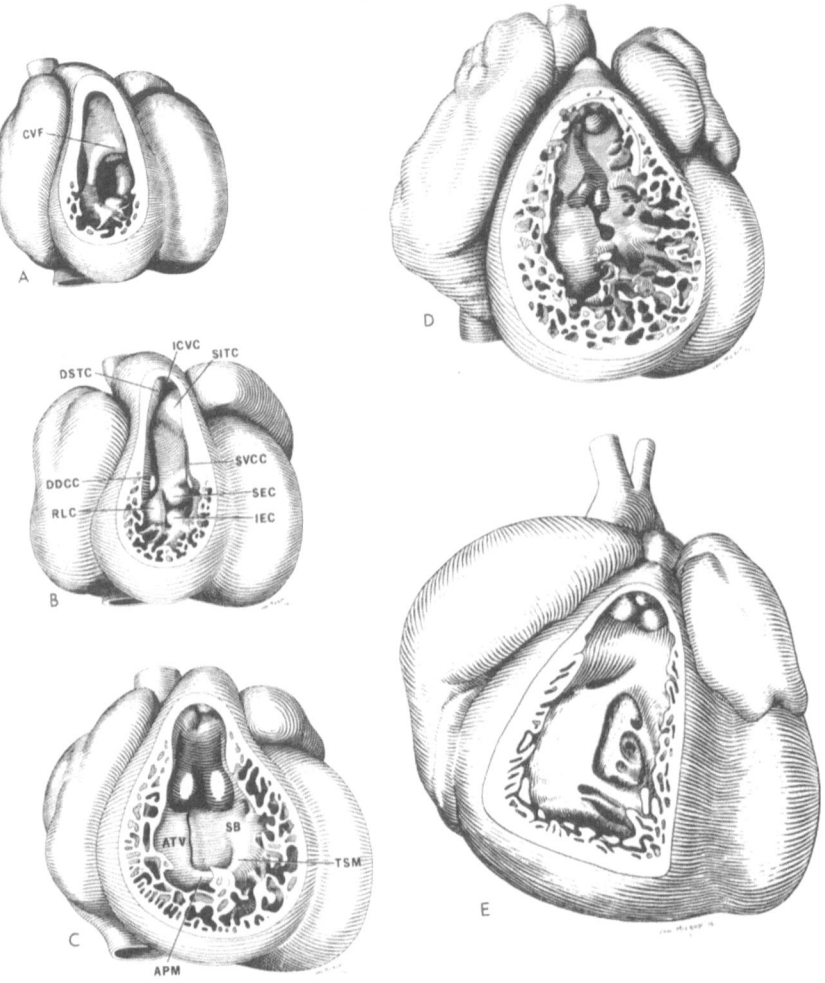

Fig. 4A-E. Normal development of the conotruncal septum in the dog. The right ventricle has been opened. **A** Heart of embryo of 4–5 mm C-R length (stage XIII), **B** 7-mm (stage XV), **C** 14-mm (stage XVIII), **D** 19-mm (stage XX). Conal cushions and conal septum are shaded darker. **E** 41-mm conal septal tissue is no longer visible. *APM* anterior papillary muscle. *ATV* anterior tricuspid cusp, *CVF* conoventricular fold, *DDCC* dextrodorsal conal cushion, *DSTC* dextrosuperior truncal cushion, *ICVC* intercalated valve cushion, *IEC* inferior endocardial cushion, *RLC* right lateral cushion, *SB* septal band, *SEC* superior endocardial cushion, *SITC* sinistroinferior truncal cushion, *SVCC* sinistroventral conal cushion, *TSM* trabecula septomarginalis. (From Van Mierop LHS et al. (1977) Hereditary conotruncal septal defects in keeshond dogs: Embryologic studies. Am J Cardiol 49: 936–950)

Meanwhile, the atrioventricular canal has enlarged to the right while the growing endocardial cushions project progressively into the lumen. In embryos of about 10 mm C-R length the major cushions reach each other and fuse, resulting in complete division of the canal into right and left atrioventricular ostia (Fig. 4). At the same time the cushions also bend, and after fusion they eventually form an arch whose concavity is directed anteriorly towards the left ventricle and whose convexity is directed posteriorly towards the atria. The free margin of the atrial septal primum meets the convex atrial side of the fused endocardial cushions about midway between the extremities and fuses with the cushions. The portion of the cushions to the left of the septum primum becomes part of the anterior or aortic cusp of the mitral valve, and therefore does not participate in the formation of the cardiac septum.

The right half of the fused endocardial cushions assumes a more sagittal position in about the same plane as the muscular interventricular septum. The communication still remaining between the right and left ventricles, the secondary interventricular foramen, is now bordered inferiorly and anteriorly by the muscular ventricular septum, posteriorly by the right extremity of the fused endocardial cushions and superiorly by the conal septum. The plane of the secondary interventricular foramen therefore, inclines somewhat to the right, but that of the primary interventricular foramen as we have seen deviates to the left. They share, however, the top of the muscular septum as part of their inferior borders. The closure of the secondary interventricular foramen requires the participation of the embryonic conal septum.

The conus cordis

The conus cordis also is partitioned by a pair of endocardial mesenchymal masses, the conal cushions. These appear at about the same time as the atrioventricular canal cushions and a third pair of cushions in the truncus arteriosus (truncal cushions) in embryos of about 6 mm C-R length. One of the conal cushions is located on the dextrodorsal conal wall, the other on the sinistroventral wall. The former eventually terminates at the superior border of the right atrioventricular ostium and blends with the right lateral and superior cushions of the atrioventricular canal. The sinistroventral conal cushion extends downwards in an apical direction along the right side of the upper anterior part of the muscular interventricular septum and blends with the upper portion of the septal band. Completion of the conal septum divides the conus into an anterolateral and a posteromedial portion. The primitive right ventricle and the anterolateral half of the conus together form the apical and outflow portions of the definitive right ventricle. The posteromedial part of the conus becomes continuous with the primitive left ventricle by way of the enlarging primary interventricular foramen, thus forming the aortic infundibulum or vestibule and establishing the definitive left ventricle. With completion of the conal septum the originally large interventricular communication becomes much smaller and is closed by fusion of endocardial cushion tissue of the conal septum, the top of the ventricular septum and the right extremity of the superior endocardial cushion. Closure is usually complete in human embryos of about 17 mm C-R length. Initially this part of the ventricular septum is thick; only much later when the fetus is about 3 months old and when the anterior portion of the septal cusp of the tricuspid valve has been formed, does an area of variable extent becomes thin and fibrous: the interventricular part of the membranous septum. The part of the endocardial cushion arch or bay between its junction with the septum primum centrally and with the ventricular septum on the right eventually becomes much thinner forming the atrioventricular portion of the septum.

For the posterobasilar part of the ventricular septum, commonly referred to as the inlet septum, to develop normally from a condensation of retained trabeculae it is necessary that the right atrioventricular ostium occupies its normal position and develops normally [14]. If it does not, e.g. as in double inlet left ventricle where both atrioventricular valves enter the same ventricular chamber, a muscle bar, the posterior muscle bundle, still

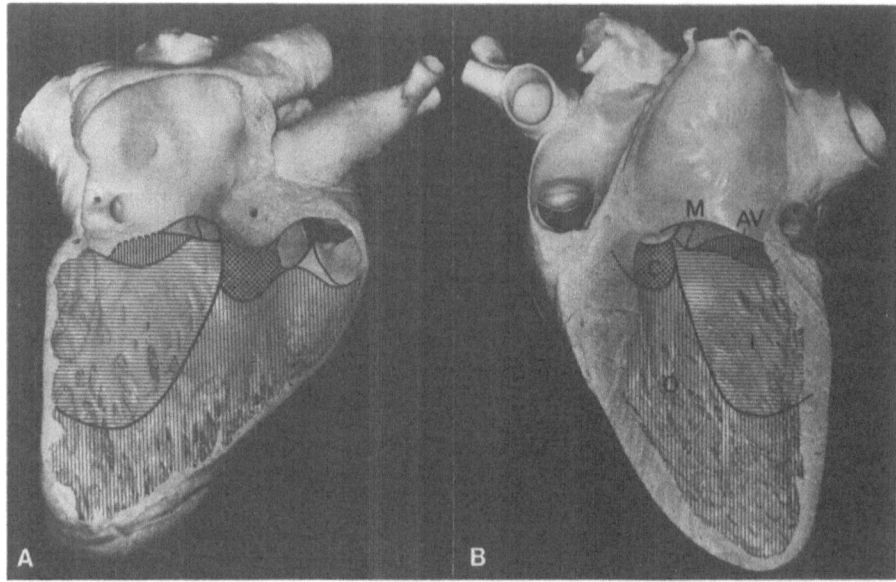

Fig. 5A, B. Normal adult ventricular septum. *AV* atrioventricular septum, *C* conal septum, *I* inlet septum, *M* membranous septum, *O* outlet septum.

develops along the posterior ventricular wall. The inlet septum therefore may develop from at least two components [15].

Discussion and comments concerning phylogeny

Most recent authors agree that the ventricular septum is derived from several components (Fig. 5). There is difference of opinion as to the extent of each of these components and their genesis as well as their nomenclature. The earliest indication of septation of the ventricular part of the early embryonic heart is the appearance of the bulboventricular fold, which is brought about by the formation of the heart loop. It is interesting that cardiac looping is a phylogenetically very old process and a well developed bulboventricular fold is already present in the shark heart [21]. As in the early embryonic heart, the ventricular portion of the shark heart is divided by the bulboventricular fold into a left sided component which receives the single atrioventricular canal and a right sided component from which the arterial trunk arises.

The anteroapical portion of the muscular ventricular septum, including the trabecula septomarginalis, is continuous with the bulboventricular fold and is considered by Wenink to be part of it [7]. This part of the septum also is phylogenetically quite ancient and is represented in the reptilian heart by the horizontal septum (horizontal in position only because reptiles generally live their lives in the prone position), also known by the older German term "Muskelleiste". Recent studies support the view that the reptilian horizontal septum is homologous with the anteroapical part of the mammalian ventricular septum, including the trabeculae septomarginalis [12]. The posterobasilar or inlet portion of the ventricular septum is probably homologous with the vertical septum, the only one of a number of sagittal septa present in amphibian and lower reptilian hearts which is retained in higher vertebrates (the others being broken up into trabeculae and papillary muscles). In Crocodilia, as in birds and mammals, it forms part of a closed ventricular septum.

Phylogenetically the youngest part of the ventricular septum to appear on the evolutionary scene and the one that develops last is the part which separates the right and left ventricular outflow tracts, i.e. the part just below the aortic and pulmonary valves. It is present only in mammals and birds. Even though in Crocodilia the ventricular septum is also complete and closed this upper portion of the septum in Crocodilia is not homologous to that in mammals, since it occupies a different position, below the right and left aortic valves rather than below the pulmonary valve and the adjacent aortic valve.

References

1. Van Mierop LHS, Alley RD, Kausel HW, Stranahan A (1963) Pathogenesis of transposition complexes.I. Embryology of the ventricles and great arteries. Am J Cardiol 12. 216-225
2. Asami I (1969) Beitrag zur Entwicklungsgeschichte des Kammerseptums im menschlichen Herzen mit besonderer Berücksichtigung der sogenannten Bulbusdrehung. Z Anat Entwicklgesch 128: 1-17
3. Goor DA, Edwards JE, Lillehei CW (1970) The development of the interventricular septum of the human heart, correlative morphogenetic study. Chest 58: 453-467
4. Anderson RH, Wilkinson JL, Arnold R, Lubkiewicz K (1974) Morphogenesis of bulboventricular malformations. I. Considerations of embryogenesis in the normal heart. Br Heart J 36: 242-255
5. Van Mierop LHS (1979) Morphological development of the heart. In: Berne RM (ed) Handbook of physiology. Am Physiol Soc, Bethesda, pp 1-28
6. Steding G, Seidle W (1980) Contribution to the development of the heart. Part I: Normal development. Thorac Cardiovasc Surg 28: 386-409
7. Wenink ACG (1981) Development of the ventricular septum. In: Wenink ACG, Oppenheimer-Dekker A, Moulaert AJ (eds) The ventricular septum of the heart. Nijhoff. The Hague, pp 23-34
8. Wenink ACG (1981) Embryology of the ventricular septum. Separate origin of its components. Virchows Arch [A] 390: 71-79
9. De la Cruz MV, Gimenez-Ribotta M, Saravalli O, Cayre R (1983) The contribution of the inferior endocardial cushion of the atrioventricular canal to cardiac septation and to the development of the atrioventricular valves: Study in the chick embryo. Am J Anat 166: 63-72
10. Grant RP (1962) Embryology of ventricular flow pathways in man. Circulation 25: 756-779
11. Davis CL (1924) The cardiac jelly of the chick embryo. Anat Rec 27: 201-202
12. Van Mierop LHS, Kutsche LM (1981) Comparative anatomy of the ventricular septum. In: Wenink ACG, Oppenheimer-Dekker A, Moulaert AJ (eds) The ventricular septum of the heart. Nijhoff, The Hague, pp 35-46
13. Moulaert AJ, Oppenheimer-Dekker A (1976) Anterolateral muscle bundle of the left ventricle, bulboventricular flange and subaortic stenosis. Am J Cardiol 37: 78-81
14. Van Mierop LHS (1979) Embryology of the univentricular heart. Herz 4: 78-85
15. Gittenberger-de Groot AC, Wenink ACG (1981) The ventricular septum in hearts with a stradding tricuspid valve. In: Wenink ACG, Oppenheimer-Dekker A, Moulaert AJ (eds) The ventricular septum of the heart. Nijhoff, The Hague, pp 175-183

Classification of ventricular septal defects
— A matter of precision*

Anton E. Becker and Robert H. Anderson

The classification of ventricular septal defects remains a contentious subject [1–6]. Hence, various authors will use different terms to describe septal defects. Regrettably, some of these terms lack precision in describing the anatomy and, thus, may give rise to different interpretations. This becomes particularly important when geographical differences in the distribution of various types of ventricular septal defects are considered.

The use of the term subpulmonic ventricular septal defect may serve as an example.

Classification of ventricular septal defects

The classification, as we advocate it [5], is based on the identification of the precise site of the defect as it relates to the membranous septum. Thus, two major groups are distinguished, viz. perimembranous and muscular ventricular septal defects (Fig. 1).

Perimembranous ventricular septal defects all share in common that the membranous septum, or its remnant, borders on the defect. This particular feature has important clinical spinoffs. Firstly, by nature of its anatomy the membranous septum is situated immediately underneath the aorta. Defects in this particular position, therefore, will by necessity be located underneath the aorta and, hence, are subaortic. The second important point is that the position of the atrioventricular conduction bundle, as it penetrates the fibrous annulus separating atrial from ventricular myocardium, closely relates to the membranous septum. Consequently, all perimembranous defects will have an intimate relationship with the atrioventricular bundle.

Perimembranous ventricular septal defects may extend predominantly into the inlet part of the ventricular septum, the trabecular part, or its outlet part. This extent also has clinical relevance, particularly with respect to the precise position of the atrioventricular conduction bundle. In inlet perimembranous defects, the atrioventricular bundle usually will take a relatively long course along the free edge of the defect, whereas in outlet perimembranous defects the area where the bundle is exposed is usually limited. Moreover, in case of outlet extension the aortic root is more intimately related to the defect than in hearts with an inlet perimembranous defect.

Muscular ventricular septal defects are per definition always completely surrounded by muscle. Their classification is completed by indicating their precise position in the ventricular septum, as indicated by the terms inlet, trabecular, and outlet. Muscular ventri-

---

* This paper appeared in Heart and Vessels Vol. 1, No. 1(1985).

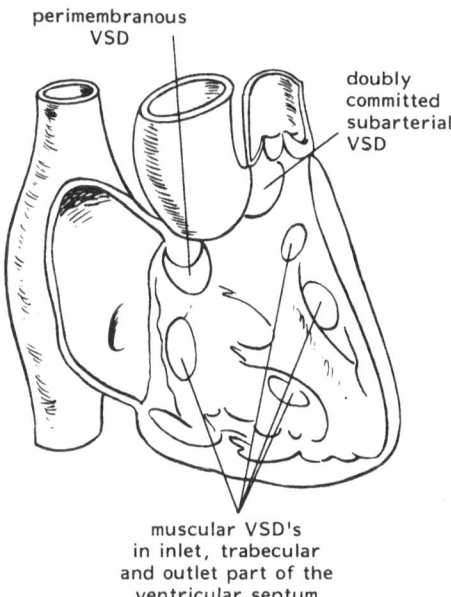

perimembranous
VSD

doubly
committed
subarterial
VSD

muscular VSD's
in inlet, trabecular
and outlet part of the
ventricular septum

Fig. 1. Schematic drawing of the basic types of ventricular septal defects. The doubly committed subarterial VSD has the valve rings of the aorta and pulmonary trunk in its roof. The extent towards the membranous septum may vary. (From Gussenhoven WJ, Becker AE (1983) Congenital heart disease. Morphologic echo-cardiographic correlations. Churchill Living-stone, Edinburgh)

cular septal defects have no direct relationship with the atrioventricular conduction bundle.

It follows from this classification that the outlet part of the ventricular septum may contain defects completely enclosed by myocardium, muscular outlet defects, and defects that may extend to the membranous septum perimembranous outlet defects. Both types of defects are "subpulmonic." However, in both types the defect is still separated from the pulmonary valve ring by a rim of muscle. Therefore, the classification [5] caters for a third type of ventricular septal defect, which has the pulmonary and aortic valve rings in its roof. These defects are called doubly committed subarterial (Fig. 1). It is important, in this respect, to emphasize that a defect which carries only the pulmonary valve ring in its roof does not exist. In the normal heart, the pulmonary valve ring is in a more cephalic position than the aortic valve ring. In case of a defect in immediate subpulmonic location, both aortic and pulmonary valve rings have to be at the same level and, hence, the defect will always be underneath both arterial rings. The only aspect that may vary is the degree in which both valve rings are committed to the roof of the defect.

In some cases of a doubly committed subarterial defect, the defect may extend to the area of the membranous septum and thus may become perimembranous. In other doubly committed defects, a bar of muscle, which may vary considerably in size, separates the defect from the membranous area. In other words, the doubly committed subarterial type of defect can be subdivided into a perimembranous variety and a type in which part of the outlet septum is present.

Finally, a so-called malalignment type ventricular septal defect is recognized, in which part of the ventricular septum (usually the outlet part) is not in alignment with the other parts, thus creating a defect. This type of defect may also be subclassified into a peri-membranous and a muscular variety, with all implications previously outlined.

Discussion

The classification of ventricular septal defects should serve a practical goal. From a hemodynamic point of view, the size of the defect is much more important than its precise position. On the other hand, the position may be considered important with respect to aspects such as aortic valve prolapse and spontaneous closure. The classification advocated in this paper is particularly tailored for the needs of the surgeon [7, 8], but gives important information also with respect to other aspects. The most important point is that defects in the ventricular septum can be described in unambiguous fashion.

As outlined in the previous paragraph, the term "subpulmonic ventricular septal defect" is imprecise. Indeed, any type of ventricular septal defect positioned in the outlet part of the ventricular septum may be termed "subpulmonic," whether basically perimembranous or muscular. Moreover, the term may give rise to the misunderstanding that a defect in the immediate subpulmonic area is solely confined to the pulmonary valve ring [6]. This is not the case since the anatomy dictates that all defects that have the pulmonary valve ring in the roof will be doubly committed subarterial rather than solely subpulmonic. This particular type of outlet defect may then be so large as to extend to the membranous septum or may be partially muscular.

Hence, a defect classified as "subpulmonic" needs extensive further specification before it becomes a meaningful term. The need for such precision becomes particularly important since "subpulmonic ventricular septal defects" have been reported to occur with a higher incidence in Japan [9] and in South America [10] than in the United States of America and Western European countries.

A rose by any other name would smell as sweet, but nevertheless roses are most precisely catalogued.

References

1. Becu LM, Fontana RS, DuShane KW, Kirklin JW, Burchell HB, Edwards JE (1956) Anatomic and pathologic studies in ventricular septal defect. Circulation 14: 349-364
2. Warden HE, DeWall RA, Cohen M, Varco RL, Lillehei CW (1957) A surgical-pathologic classification for isolated ventricular septal defects and for those in Fallot's tetralogy based on observations made on 120 patients during repair under direct vision. J Thorac Cardiovasc Surg 33: 21-44
3. Neufeld HN, Titus JL, DuShane JW, Burchell HB, Edwards JE (1961) Isolated ventricular septal defect of the persistent common atrioventricular canal type. Circulation 23: 685-696
4. Goor DA, Lillehei CW, Rees R, Edwards JE (1970). Isolated ventricular septal defect: Development basis for various types and presentation of classification. Chest 58: 468-482
5. Soto B, Becker AE, Lie JT, Moulaert A, Anderson RH (1980) Classification of ventricular septal defects. Br Heart J 43: 332-343
6. Capelli M, Andrade JL, Somerville J (1983) Classification of the site of ventricular septal defect by 2-dimensional echocardiography. Am J Cardiol 51: 1474-1480
7. Milo S, Ho SY, Wilkinson JL, Anderson RH (1980) The surgical anatomy and atrioventricular conduction tissues of hearts with isolated ventricular septal defects. J Thorac Cardiovasc Surg 79: 244-255
8. Kurosawa H, Becker AE (1984) Modification of the precise relationship of the atrioventricular conduction bundle to the margins of the ventricular septal defects by the trabecula septomarginalis. J Thorac Cardiovasc Surg 87: 605-615
9. Ando M (1974) Subpulmonary ventricular septal defect with pulmonary stenosis (Letter to the editor). Circulation 50: 412
10. Neirotti R, Galindez E, Kreutzer G, Coronel AR, Pedeini M, Becu L (1978) Tetralogy of Fallot with subpulmonary ventricular septal defect. Ann Thorac Surg 25: 51-56

Pathological anatomy of ventricular septal defect associated with aortic valve prolapse and regurgitation*

Masahiko Ando and Atsuyoshi Takao

Aortic regurgitation (AR) due to a prolapsed aortic cusp(prolapsing AR) is one of the most common complications seen in Japanese patients with ventricular septal defect (VSD) [1, 2]. This fact is clearly demonstrated in that well-trained pediatric cardiologists in Japan usually expect to find this condition in almost every child presenting with VSD, especially if the patient has a less than moderate defect. Many clinicians who deal with the condition now consider that prolapsing aortic valve associated with VSD might be specific to Japanese or Oriental people.

Although several reports on the pathological anatomy have been published [3, 7], they usually deal with limited numbers of cases. The pathogenetic mechanism of the syndrome is not yet fully understood. The purpose of this report is to clarify the underlying pathogenetic morphology of this syndrome based upon autopsy-proven Japanese cases and to consider the clinical implications of the findings for better management of the condition.

Materials and methods

The material basis of this study consisted of 61 hearts with VSD and prolapsing aortic valve with or without AR (Table 1). These were found among 201 heart specimens with 202 VSD. All these hearts were from the collection of the Heart Institute of Japan, which consists of 1700 specimens with congenital heart disease (CHD). Therefore, VSD associated with prolapsing aortic valve amounts to 4% of all autopsy-proven cases of CHD.

The cases were divided into three groups according to the complications: Group 1, those with prolapsed aortic valve (32 cases); group 2, those with prolapsed aortic valve and AR (20 cases); and group 3, those with a significant sinus of Valsalva aneurysm in addition to the complications seen in group 2 (nine cases).

Eighty-five percent (52/61) of the hearts were from autopsy specimens obtained before 1973. In that year, the management of the condition was tentatively established at our institute [1, 5–7], and since then we have experienced only few autopsy cases with prolapsing AR.

The cause of death was related to cardiac surgery in two-thirds of the cases (Table 1). Medical death was due mainly to congestive heart failure in group 1. In this group, half of the patients were under 3 years of age and had a more than moderate VSD with a massive left-to-right shunt. Prolapsed aortic valve in group 1 cases was mainly diagnosed after post-

---

*This paper appeared in Heart and Vessels Vol. 2, No. 2 (1986).

Table 1. VSD with prolapsing aortic valve. Subgrouping according to complications and salient clinical profiles

	No. of cases	Male	Female	Age range (median)	Cause of death Surgical	Cause of death Medical
Prolapsed AoV	32	16	14	1 mo – 14 yrs (3 yrs)	20	12 (CHF)
Prolapsed AoV + AR	20	11	9	4 yrs – 34 yrs (16 yrs)	19	1 (IE)
Valsalva aneurysm	9	6	3	13 yrs – 60 yrs (25 yrs)	3	6 (rupture, IE)
Total	61	33	26		42	19

Numbers in each column shows number of patients observed

mortem examination. In groups 2 and 3, medical death was due to ruptured aneurysm of the sinus of Valsalva in five cases and to infective endocarditis in two (Table 1).

There was a preponderance of males (Table 1), as has been reported in the literature [4, 7, 10, 15]. Group 1 with prolapsing aortic valve was mainly seen during infancy (median age, 3 years). Group 2 with AR was distributed from late childhood to young adulthood (median age, 16 years). Group 3 with Valsalva aneurysm was observed after adolescence (median age, 25 years). The age distribution among each group suggests the progression of the condition in this order (Table 1) [15]. The Valsalva aneurysm seen in group 3 cases is considered to be a complication of the condition seen in group 2 cases; these two groups will, therefore, be discussed together.

These 61 hearts were examined with special reference to the type of septal alignment, location and size of the defect, its relation to the aortic valve, and abnormalities of the aortic valve and sinus of Valsalva wall.

Anatomical types of isolated VSD

The classification of the anatomical types was done conventionally according to the location of the defect [11, 14]. There are three developmental components in the ventricular septum, i.e., the infundibular and muscular sinus septa and, between the two, the membranous septum. The sinus septum consists of two parts — the inflow smooth and apical trabecular septa [12].

VSD can occur within each septal component and along their junctions. The cases of the former type were usually of a simple punched hole in a septal component with normal septal alignment (simple punched-hole type VSD). The same morphology can be present in the latter type, which involves the junction of two adjoining septa. However, a significant number of the latter cases at the ventricular outflow tract were due to a malalignment of the adjacent septa, involving the infundibuloventricular or infundibulotruncal junction. There are two kinds of malalignment-type VSD. In Eisenmenger-type VSD [2, 13], the infundibular or truncal septum deviates anteriorly away from the left ventricular outflow tract, but there is no infundibular stenosis. In coarctation-type VSD [2], the septum deviates posteriorly close to the mitral valve, inducing variable degrees of subaortic narrowing and frequent association with coarctation or interruption of the aorta.

Table 2. Racial difference in the location of isolated VSD

Type of VSD	HIJ Series (Japanese)		Soto's series (mainly Caucasian)	
	Percentage	No.	Percentage	No.
Infundibular VSD	63	128	25	57
Subarterial IVSD	30	60	5	12
Muscular IVSD	8	16	1	3
Perimembranous IVSD	23	47	19	42
Total IVSD	2	5	—	—
Perimembranous trabecular VSD	21	43	25	56
Perimembranous inlet VSD	12	24	25	55
Muscular VSD	4	7	25	55
Total		202		223

Table 2. Racial comparison in relative frequencies of anatomic types according to the location of isolated VSD was performed between Japanese and Caucasian autopsy series. Infundibular VSD(IVSD) is more than twice as common in Japanese as in Caucasians. Subarterial doubly committed or subpulmonic IVSD, which is the form most often associated with prolapsing AR, is especially prevalent in the Japanese series. In contract, muscular VSD is much more common in the Caucasian than in the Japanese series. P < 0.02

In the classification shown in Table 2, only the location of the defect could be considered for a comparison of racial difference in the anatomical type of VSD, because all the reported series of Caucasians [11, 14] included only the location of the defects. However, in viewing the anatomical types of isolated VSD, we should always consider the presence or absence of septal malalignment, i.e., simple punched-hole, Eisenmenger and coarctation types (Fig. 1), in addition to the location of the VSD, as this feature has considerable clinical significance [2].

Relative incidence of VSD

As all the 61 hearts with this condition showed an infundibular VSD (IVSD) closely related to the aortic valve and because of the relative rarity of the condition in reported series from other countries [3, 4, 8-10], we updated the relative incidences of each anatomical type of isolated VSD. We then compared these figures with those of a recent paper by Soto et al. [11], which was the outcome of a joint study among institutions in the United States and Europe (Table 2). Sixty-three percent or 128 of 202 VSD found in 201 hearts were infundibular in the Japanese series. However, only 25% showed IVSD in the Caucasian series. A remarkable increase in IVSD, especially of the subpulmonic or subarterial type, in Japanese may correspond well with the high incidence of VSD associated with AR in our country, whereas VSD at the inflow tract are much more common in Caucasians. These results reconfirm the racial difference in the relative incidence of the anatomical types of uncomplicated VSD, which we have reported previously [2, 5].

Results

Location of the VSD

Concerning the location of the defect, subpulmonic or subarterial doubly committed IVSD is the most common site for developing a prolapsed aortic valve (Table 3). In this type of IVSD, 72% showed a prolapsed aortic valve with or without AR. Other types of infundibular VSD, i.e., muscular, perimembranous, or total IVSD, associated with the condition are seen at a much lower frequency, i.e., 20%–31% of each type.

In the autopsy group, 30% of all VSD, or 48% of IVSD, had a prolapsed aortic valve, and half of them had developed AR.

Table 3. Location of VSD and prolapsing aortic valve

Type of VSD	All VSD Cases		Prolapsed Ao valve No. of cases	Prolapsed AoV with AR No. of cases	Total (Pr. AoV $\bar{C}/\bar{S}$ AR)	
	No.	Percentage			No. of cases	Percentage
Subarterial IVSD	60	30	19	24	43	72
Muscular IVSD	16	8	3	2	5	31
Perimembranous IVSD	47	23	9	3	12	25
Total IVSD	5	2	1	0	1	20
Perimembranous VSD (trabecular, inlet)	67	33	0	0	0	0
Muscular VSD	7	4	0	0	0	0
Total	202	100	32	29	61	30

The relative incidence of prolapsed aortic valve and of prolapsing AR are shown in each type of VSD in which only location of the defect is considered. Prolapsing aortic valve with or without AR is seen only in VSD at the infundibular septum (IVSD).

	Normal	Eisenmenger Type	Coarc Type	Total
Subarterial I VSD				Pr + AR 24 Pr 18
Muscular I VSD				Pr + AR 2 Pr 4
Perimembranous I VSD				Pr + AR 3 Pr 9
Total I VSD				Pr 1
Total	Pr + AR 27 Pr 23	Pr + AR 2 Pr 8	Pr 1	Pr + Ar 29 Pr 32

: Pr + AR   : Pr
: Aneurysm   : Normal Ao V

Fig. 1. Septal alignment and VSD with prolapsing aortic valve. Incidence of prolapsing aortic valve with or without AR is shown according to the type of septal alignment in addition to the location of IVSD. *Normal:* a simple punched-hole IVSD with normal septal alignment, *Eisenmenger Type:* VSD in which the infundibular or truncal septum is deviated anteriorly away from the left ventricular outflow tract but without infundibular obstruction, *Coarc Type:* VSD in which the infundibular or truncal septum is deviated posteriorly close to the mitral valve, inducing variable degrees of subaortic narrowing. Prolapsing aortic valve with or without AR is common in simple punched-hole type IVSD, being the most common (100%) in those with subarterial doubly committed IVSD; it is rather rare in cases with malalignment-type IVSD. *AoV:* aorticc valve, *Pr:* prolapsed aortic valve

The type of septal alignment

Figure 1 shows the occurrence of prolapsing AR in relation to the presence or absence of septal malalignment. As mentioned previously, there are three types of IVSD according to the kind of septal alignment, i.e., simple punched-hole type, Eisenmenger-type, and coarctation-type VSD. The latter two are malalignment-type VSD.

In simple punched-hole IVSD with normal septal alignment, 44% (27/62) of cases showed prolapsing AR with a large Valsalva aneurysm in nine cases, and another 37% (23/62) revealed a prolapsed aortic valve (Fig. 1). Among these IVSD, subpulmonic or subarterial IVSD is the most common site for the syndrome. All cases of this subtype developed a prolapsing aortic valve. AR was present in 60% (24/40) of them, of which eight cases (20%) showed a significant aneurysm of the sinus of Valsalva. Sixty-two percent (5/8) of muscular and 35% (5/14) of perimembranous IVSD with normal septal alignment developed a prolapsing aortic valve. Some of the cases suffered from AR with or without aneurysm formation (Fig. 1).

In contrast to the cases with the simple punched-hole type, those with malalignment-type VSD revealed a much lower frequency. Ten of forty cases (25%) with Eisenmenger-type and one of twenty-five (4%) with coarctation-type IVSD showed a prolapsed aortic valve with or without AR. Among them, 23% (7/30) of the cases with perimembranous IVSD of the Eisenmenger type revealed aortic valve prolapse and two of them developed AR.

Therefore, the common form associated with prolapsing AR is simple punched-hole IVSD, and the rare form is malalignment-type IVSD. The anatomical findings of both forms are discussed below.

Simple punched-hole type IVSD

This is the common form of IVSD associated with a prolapsed aortic valve and AR. In this type, the VSD is a simple muscular defect in any portion of the infundibular septum between the pulmonary valve above and the membranous septum below. Three subtypes can be distinguished according to the location of the defect (Fig. 2). The most common site of IVSD with prolapsing AR is the subpulmonic or subarterial doubly committed position. There are several common anatomical findings noted in these IVSD. There is no septal malalignment. The aortic valve position is completely normal. The defect is a simple muscular defect in a portion of the infundibular septum along the aortic annulus. Therefore, the annulus and sinus of Valsalva wall of the right coronary cusp, which are normally firmly supported by the septum, become exposed in the defect and poorly supported (Fig. 3). The exposed sinus of Valsalva wall is usually covered by a thin fibrous tissue (Fig. 3A, C), which appears to be a remnant of the infundibular septum. This anatomical feature suggests that in early development, the conus cushions once fused to form the septum and the aortic valve then descended normally upon it, but the septum was not muscularized later, resulting in a simple punched-hole defect. This type of VSD has three aspects in one defect: a relatively large oval-shaped muscular defect, the original VSD which has a triangular or half-moon shape with the right border formed by the denuded annulus and sinus of Valsalva wall, and a functioning VSD which has a crescent-moon to slitlike shape or is closed in rare cases according to the degree of the prolapsing aortic valve (Fig. 3).

In the majority (21/23) of the cases with a prolapsing aortic valve only (Fig. 1), there was a more than moderate (i.e., defect over half the aortic valve area) muscular defect, and the functioning VSD in these cases was still moderate in 16 of them. Among the 27 cases which had developed AR, 17 had a more than moderate muscular defect, but the

Subarterial IVSD

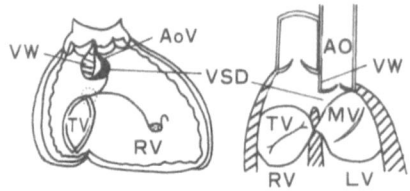

Muscular IVSD

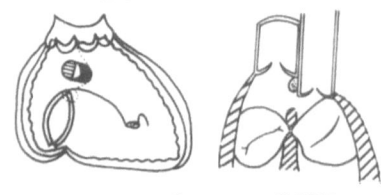

Perimembranous IVSD

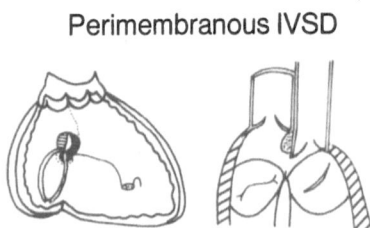

Fig. 2. Anatomical types of simple punched-hole IVSD. The right ventricular view is shown on the *left*; on the *right*, a schematic frontal projection of the cut surface perpendicular to each septal component is shown. There are three subtypes according to the location of the defect. In these IVSD, infundibular septal alignment is normal (cf. Fig. 1), and part of the right sinus of Valsalva wall and of the aortic valvular annulus are denuded in the VSD, resulting in very weak valvular support but with a normal aortic valve and position. *VW* wall of sinus of Valsalva of aortic valve, *AoV* aortic valve, *RV* right ventricle, *LV* left ventricle, *TV* tricuspid valve, *MV* mitral valve.

functioning VSD in these cases was slitlike in fifteen and closed in two cases. Bicuspid aortic valve (two cases) and Valsalva wall deformity (one case) were rare in these 50 cases of simple punched-hole IVSD with this syndrome.

The unsupported portion of the right coronary cusp moves toward the noncoronary cusp in relation to the location of the IVSD. In two of five cases with perimembranous IVSD, a small part of the noncoronary cusp also prolapsed into the VSD with the right coronary cusp. The unsupported area was 20%–70% of the right coronary annulus, depending upon the size of the muscular defect, irrespective of the location of the defect with a mean area of 40%. In any subtype of IVSD, there was no significant difference in the dimension of the unsupported part of the cusp between those with prolapsed aortic valve only and those which had developed AR.

Several examples of each subtype of simple punched-hole IVSD are illustrated in Figs. 3–8.

Malalignment-type IVSD

In Eisenmenger-type VSD, 10 of the 40 cases (25%) had a prolapsed aortic valve, and two of them which had a perimembranous IVSD developed AR (Fig. 1). In coarctation-type IVSD, only one of 25 cases (4%) showed a prolapsing aortic valve. It was found that this type of IVSD rarely developed prolapsing AR.

There are several common anatomical findings in these 11 cases (Table 4). The septal malalignment is less than moderate and dextroposition (or levoposition) is mild to moderate. The size of the VSD is usually moderate or less. All hearts have some kind of aortic valve and/or sinus of Valsalva anomaly. Four of eleven cases (36%) had a bicuspid aortic

Table 4. Anatomical findings of malalignment-type IVSD with prolapsing aortic valve with or without AR

Finding	No. of cases
Mild dextroposition (or levoposition) of Ao	11/11
Less than moderate VSD	11/11
Ao valve and sinus of Valsalva wall deformities	11/11
Bicuspid Ao valve	
(low coronary comm)	4/11
Uneven division of Ao cusps	6/11
Deformed sinus of Valsalva wall	
(due to malalignment)	7/11
Part of Ao cusps are exposed in VSD	11/11

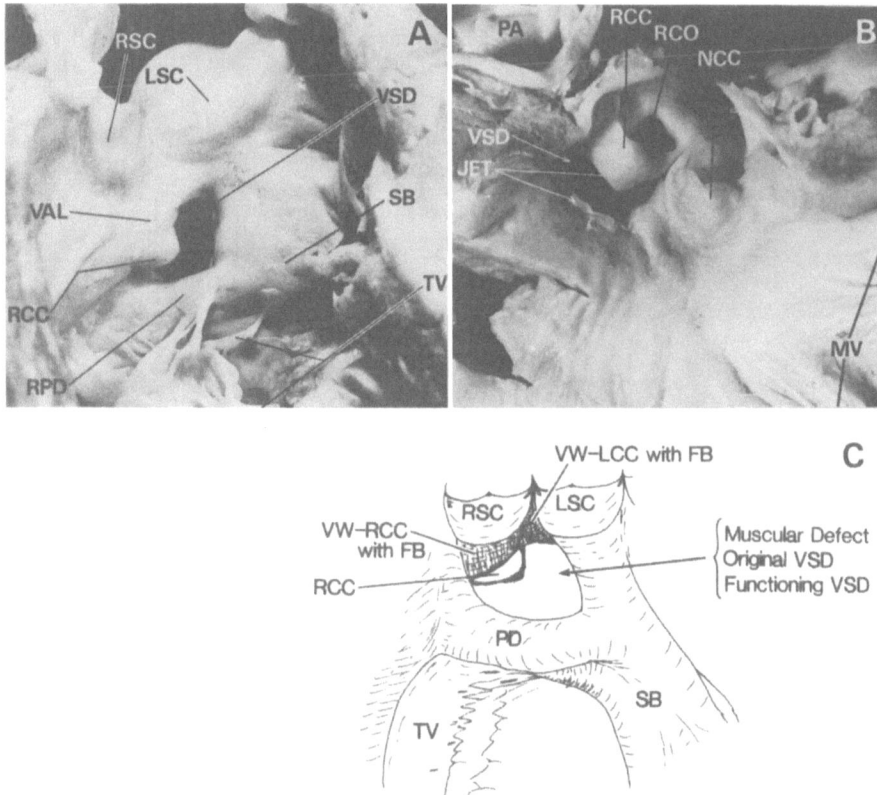

Fig. 3 A-C. Subarterial IVSD of simple punched-hole type with prolapsing aortic valve. **A** Right ventricular view. The muscular defect is immediately subpulmonic. Part of the sinus of Valsalva wall (*VAL*) and of the annulus of the right coronary cusp (*RCC*) are denuded on the right half of the muscular defect, and their support is weak. The VSD is partially narrowed by a prolapsing right coronary cusp. **B** Left ventricular view. The right coronary cusp (*RCC*) is mildly prolapsing with the formation of jet lesions (*JET*) but is still competent. **C** Schematic drawing of **A**. Exposed sinus of Valsalva wall (*VW*) is covered by a thin fibrous infundibular septum. There are three aspects in this type of VSD — the muscular defect, original VSD, and functioning VSD. Figure shows a 10-month-old male boy. *RSC, LSC* right, left septal cusp of pulmonary valve, *LCC* left coronary cusp, *SB* septal band, *PD* right posterior division of SB, *TV* tricuspid valve

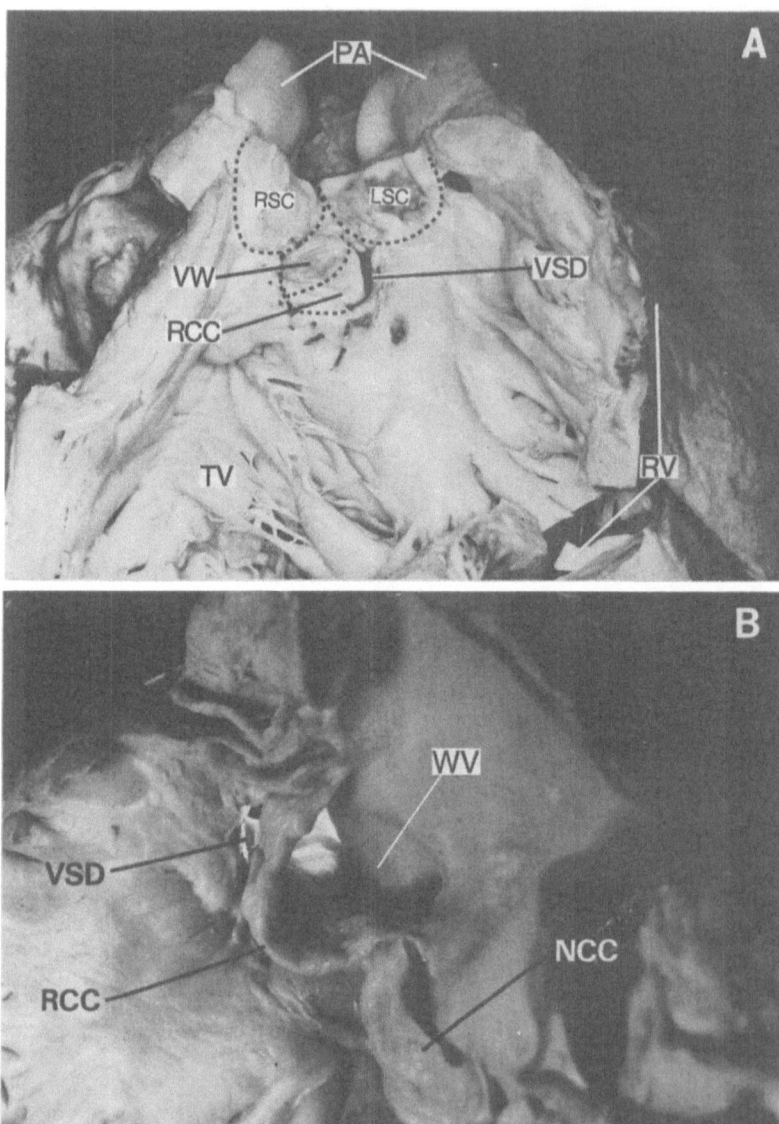

Fig. 4 A, B. Subarterial IVSD of simple punched-hole type with prolapsing AR. **A** Right ventricular view. The VSD is slitlike due to the prolapsed right coronary cusp (*RCC*), part of which has fused to the VSD rim due to jet lesions. **B** Left ventricular view. The aortic valve is severely incompetent with remarkably thickened leaflets. The prolapsed part of the right coronary cusp is transilluminated, and above it is the denuded part of the sinus of Valsalva wall (*VW*). Figure shows a 12-year-old male. Abbreviations are as in previous figures

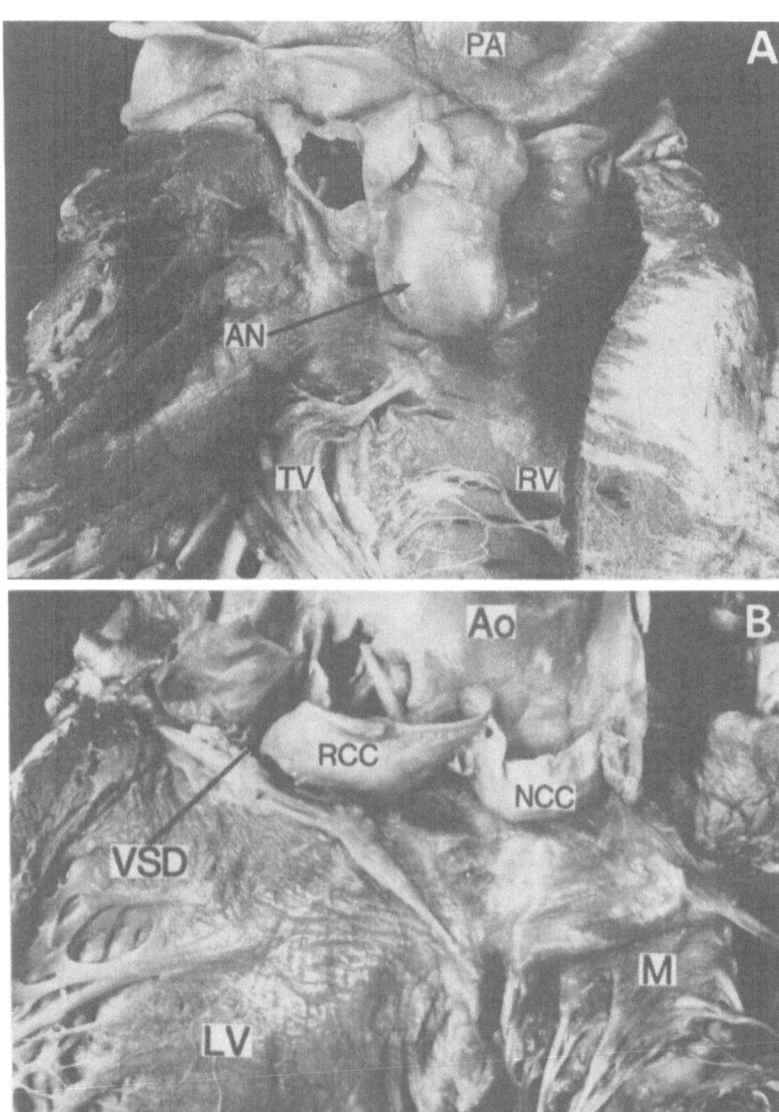

Fig. 5 A, B. Subarterial IVSD simple punched-hole type with sinus of Valsalva aneurysm. **A** Right ventricular view. A huge aneurysm of the sinus of Valsalva is present in the right ventricular outflow tract, which induces severe subpulmonic stenosis. The VSD is slitlike and closing. **B** Left ventricular view. The aortic valve angle is considerably well maintained, and only mild AR is present. It is notable that two-thirds of the cases with a significant sinus of Valsalva aneurysm formation had only mild AR. Figure shows a 25-year-old female. *AN* aneurysm of sinus of Valsalva, *M* mitral valve. Other abbreviations are as in previous figures

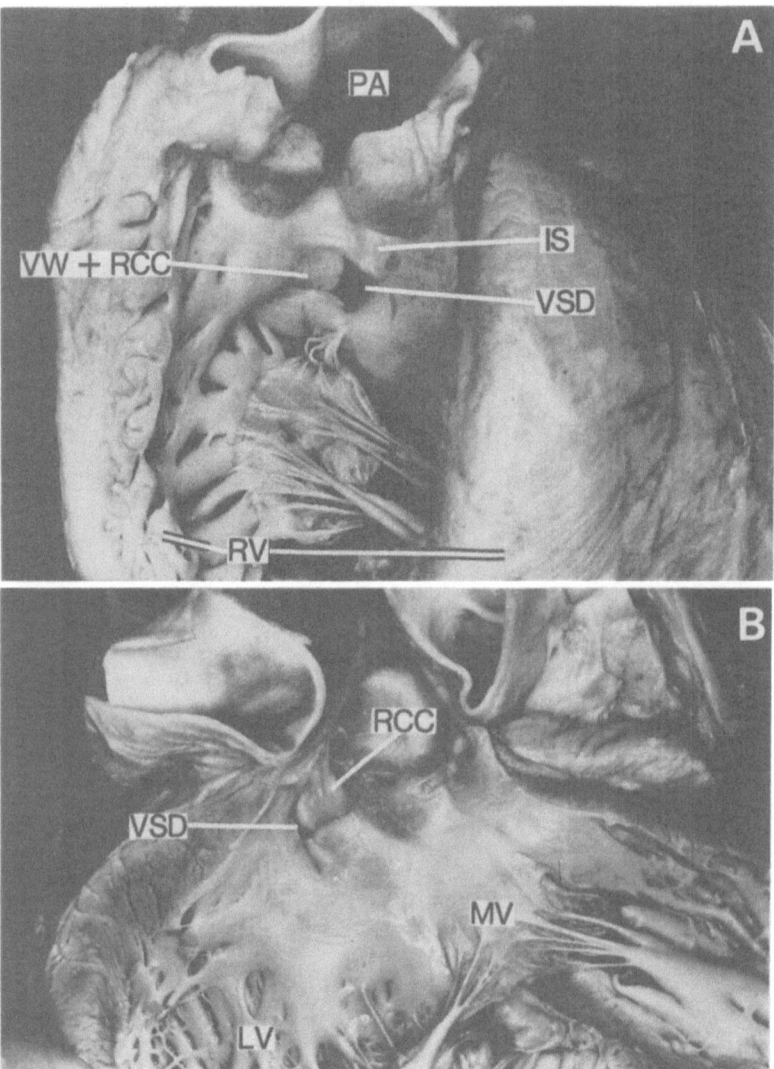

Fig. 6 A, B. Muscular IVSD of simple punched-hole type with prolapsing aortic valve. **A** Right ventricular view. The VSD is midinfundibular. Part of the sinus of Valsalva wall and right coronary annulus (*VW +* *RCC*) is denuded in the defect. The muscular infundibular septum (*IS*), which is thin and hypoplastic, intervenes between the VSD below and the pulmonary valve above. **B** Left ventricular view. The aortic valve is mildly prolapsing into the VSD. Figure shows a 2-year-old male. Abbreviations are as in previous figures

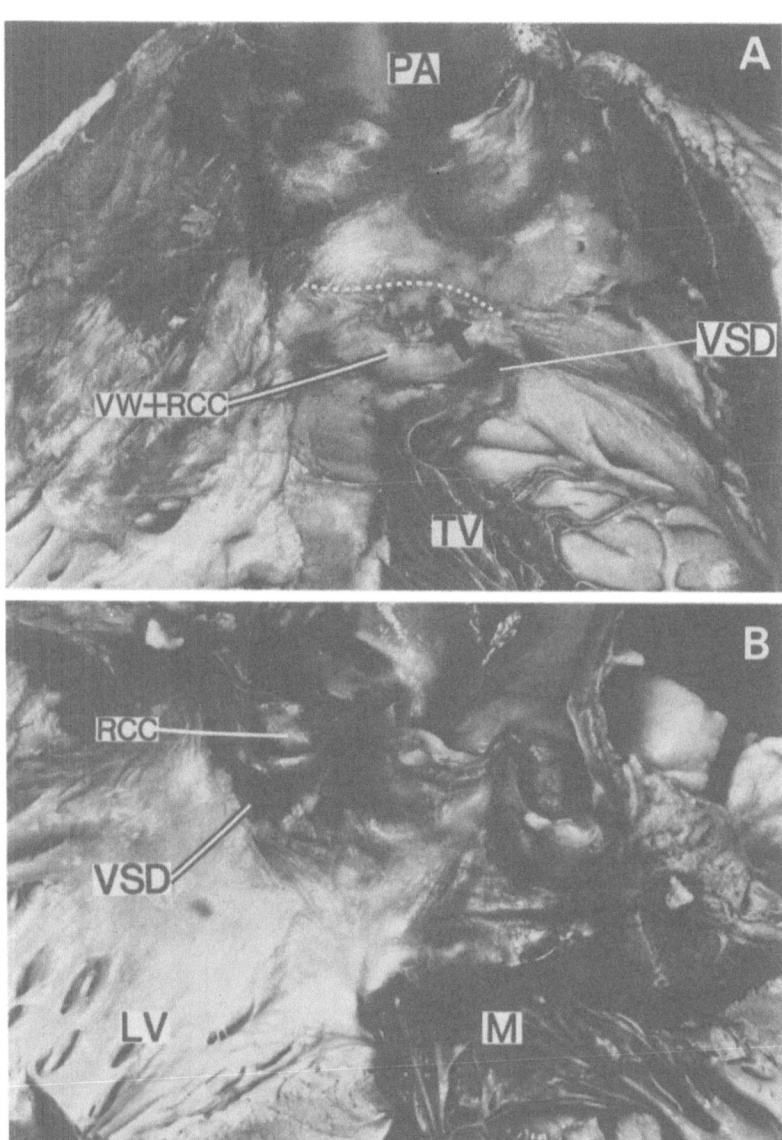

Fig. 7 A, B. Muscular IVSD of simple punched-hole type with ruptured aneurysm of sinus of Valsalva. **A** Right ventricular view. The VSD is slitlike due to the prolapsed right coronary cusp. The aneurysm originating at a weakened portion of the defective sinus of Valsalva wall is ruptured into the right ventricle (*arrow*). **B** Left ventricular view. The aortic valve is competent in this case with almost normal cusp angles and good coaptation of the cusps. Figure shows a 21-year-old male. Abbreviations are as in previous figures

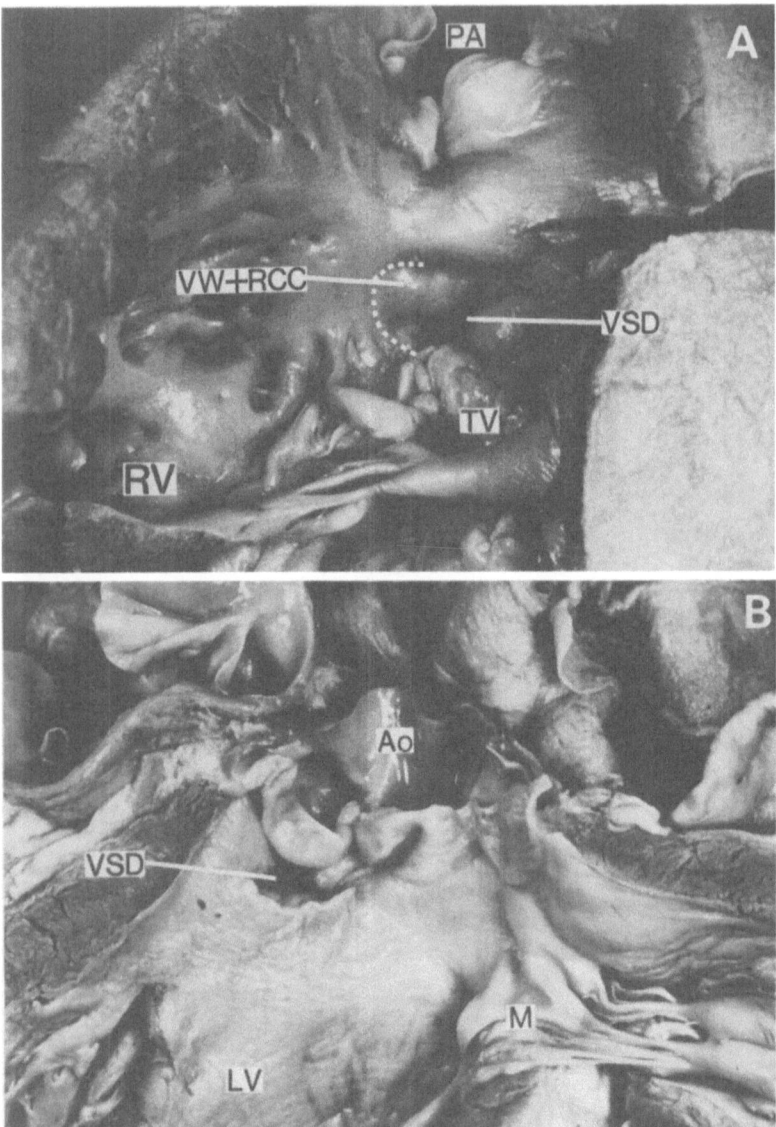

Fig. 8 A, B. Perimembranous IVSD of simple punched-hole type with prolapsing aortic valve. **A** Right ventricular view. The VSD is perimembranous with an outlet extension. Part of the right coronary sinus of Valsalva wall and the aortic annulus (*VW + RCC*) is denuded in the VSD. **B** Left ventricular view. The right coronary cusp is moderately prolapsed and mildly incompetent. Figure shows a 14-year-old female. Abbreviations are as in previous figures

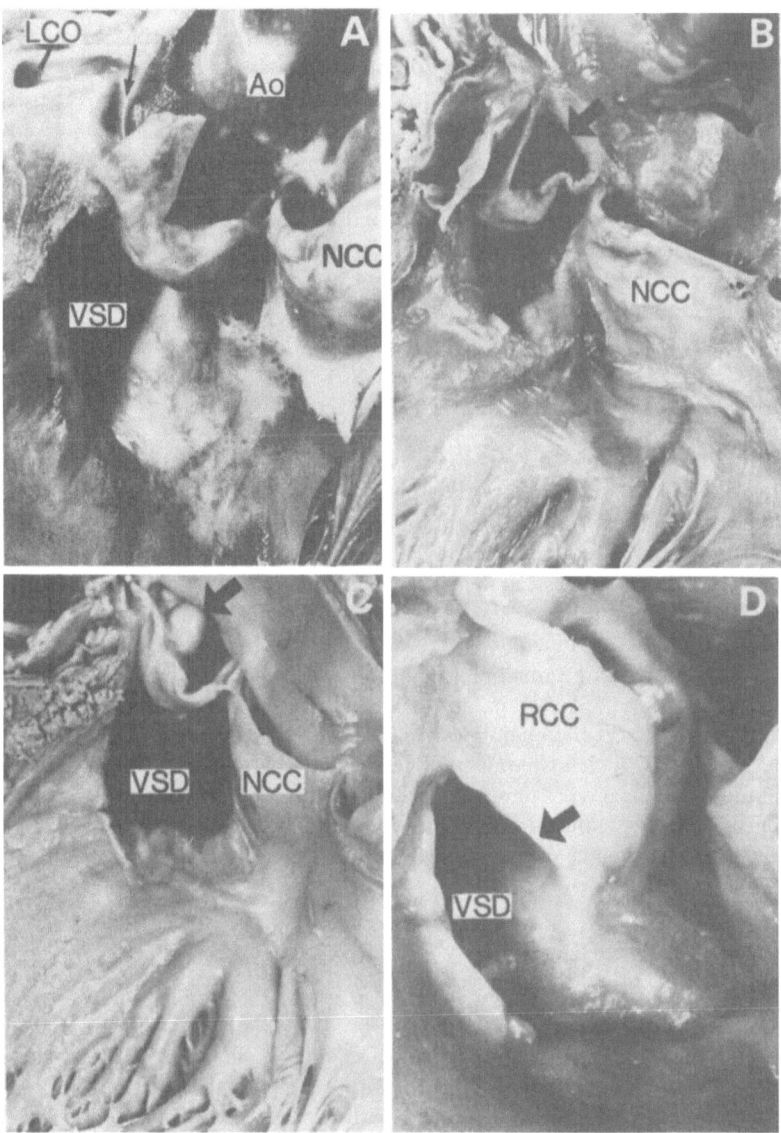

Fig. 9 A-D. Anomalies of the aortic valve and sinus of Valsalva found in cases with malalignment-type IVSD. **A** Bicuspid aortic valve due to low coronary commissure. **B** Uneven division of cusps with severe angulation of the sinus of Valsalva wall to the right. The right coronary cusp is unusually small and incompetent. **C** Deformed sinus of Valsalva wall. **D** Defective sinus of Valsalva wall in subarterial IVSD of coarctation type. Abbreviations are as in previous figures

valve due to low coronary commissure (Fig. 9A). Seven cases (64%) had a deformed sinus of Valsalva wall with severe angulation toward the right ventricular outflow tract (Fig. 9B, C). Six of these cases (55%) had uneven division of the aortic cusps, and the right coronary cusp was unusually small and often shallow (Fig. 9). In two-thirds of these cases, inherent deformities of the aortic valve and its apparatus were malignant, and development of AR might be inevitable.

In cases of malalignment-type IVSD, the aortic valve is usually well supported from below without the denuded portion of the sinus of Valsalva wall, a minority of the cases, however, have anomalies of the aortic valve and its apparatus, some of which may develop AR. These anomalies of the aortic valve and the sinus of Valsalva appear to be related to the septal malalignment of a less than moderate degree.

Discussion

In this study, we have confirmed our clinical impression that IVSD is prevalent in Japanese with isolated VSD and that a considerable number of the cases develop prolapsing AR. In Caucasian autopsy series, it is reported that IVSD is seen in 25% [11] or 28% [14] of cases of isolated VSD, and a 5% clinical incidence of AR among patients with VSD is accepted [4, 10]. In contrast, in the present Japanese autopsy series, 63% of cases with isolated VSD were infundibular, and 47% of them developed prolapsing aortic valve with or without AR. Although inherent selection of cases may exist in those included in an autopsy series, the selection probably does not differ so much between countries in hospital-based series. Moreover, such pathological studies are the most accurate method available at present to detect the anatomical variations of CHD among races. In other common forms of CHD, such as tetralogy of Fallot and coarctation-type VSD, racial differences in the anatomical types have been postulated from autopsy series [2]. If these racial differences exist, the clinical implication would be that each country should tailor the management of a particular disease according to the anatomical variant commonly found among its people.

Anatomical types of VSD with prolapsing AR

Van Praagh and McNamara [3] stated in their excellent anatomical study on this syndrome that there were two types — subcristal VSD and subpulmonic VSD. The former had herniation of the right and/or noncoronary cusp into the VSD due to a bicuspid valve and showed a septal malalignment with frequent association with infundibular pulmonary stenosis; the latter developed herniation of the right coronary cusp through the VSD due to weak valve support from below.

We are able to add several other anatomical findings from studies on Japanese autopsy specimens. There are two principal forms of IVSD: (1) Simple punched-hole IVSD with normal septal alignment and (2) malalignment IVSD, which includes Eisenmenger-type IVSD with an anteriorly deviated infundibular or truncal septum and coarctation-type IVSD with a posteriorly deviated septum. Both types — have several subtypes according to the location of the defect, i.e., subpulmonic, muscular, perimembranous and total IVSD. The common form for prolapsing AR is simple punched-hole IVSD, in which subpulmonic IVSD (subpulmonic VSD of Van Praagh's classification) constitutes 72% (24/29) of cases, and the rare form is malalignment VSD, in which perimembranous IVSD of the Eisenmenger type (subcristal VSD of Van Praagh) is the only subtype with AR in the present series and constitutes 7% (2/29) of cases (Fig. 1).

In simple punched-hole IVSD, the aortic valve is normally formed except that the annulus and a part of the sinus of Valsalva wall of the right coronary cusp, which are normally supported firmly by the infundibular septum, have become exposed in the defect and are poorly supported. The muscular defect is relatively large, but the functioning VSD is less than moderate in size with a half-moon shape below the denuded sinus of Valsalva (Fig. 3 A-C). The defect appears to become narrower in accordance with the degree of prolapse of the cusp into the defect, resulting in a crescent-moon to slitlike shape or spontaneous closure in rare cases.

In malalignment VSD, there is a VSD of moderate size with mild to moderate septal malalignment. These cases are almost always associated with intrinsic aortic valve anomalies (bicuspid or uneven division) and/or anomalies of the sinus of Valsalva (Fig. 9). In the present series, prolapsing AR associated with a malalignment VSD was only seen in two cases with perimembranous IVSD of the Eisenmenger type. However, if group 1 cases with prolapsing aortic valve only are included, which are considered to be in the prodromal stage of prolapsing AR, the whole spectrum of the syndrome can be understood (Fig. 1).

These defective aortic valves of the two forms (common and rare) are subjected to hemodynamic effects of the bloodstream.

Pathogenetic mechanism

The development of prolapsing AR appears to be due to the interaction between the above-mentioned anatomical defects and hemodynamic factors, among which the most important is the decrease of pressure in the rapid blood flow through the VSD according to Bernoulli's theorem. We have repeatedly demonstrated this interaction in angiographic studies in several previous papers [5, 6, 16]. The significance of the hemodynamic factors has been well shown by de la Cruz et al. [17] in experimentally produced IVSD in chicks. In their study, eggs incubated at a low temperature (35.83°C) showed an increase in the incidence (24.5%) of subpulmonic IVSD but without a prolapsed aortic valve when the chicks were killed on hatching. However, part of the experimental group killed after reaching adulthood showed an IVSD with a prolapsed aortic valve. This malformation is apparently acquired and is secondary to the postnatal hemodynamic effects on the inherent defect of the aortic valve, i.e., the lack of support.

The importance of the hemodynamic factors in this syndrome is evident in one case of the present series. A 15-year-old boy had a moderate subarterial IVSD of the simple punched-hole type, which had been associated with pulmonary vascular obstruction since early childhood. He had been cyanotic and died of longstanding congestive heart failure due to severe pulmonary hypertension. Autopsy revealed only mild prolapse of the aortic valve in spite of the presence of poor aortic support from below with a denuded sinus of Valsalva wall. In addition to this, the patient had a bicuspid aortic valve due to low coronary commissure, which is very rare in cases of simple punched-hole IVSD. However, if it coexists in this type of VSD, the early occurrence of prolapsing AR can be expected: The youngest patient in the present series, who developed AR at 4 years of age, had this combination. We speculate that there might have been no significant left-to-right shunting of blood through VSD during his entire life, therefore no significant hemodynamic effects nor prolapsing AR were seen in this 15-year-old boy.

In view of the above-mentioned facts, the developmental process of the prolapsing AR can be shown as in Fig. 10. During systole, especially in the early phase, the weakened aortic cusp is strongly pulled into the VSD due to the decrease of pressure in the rapid blood flow through the defect according to Bernoulli's theorem. Angiographically, this is

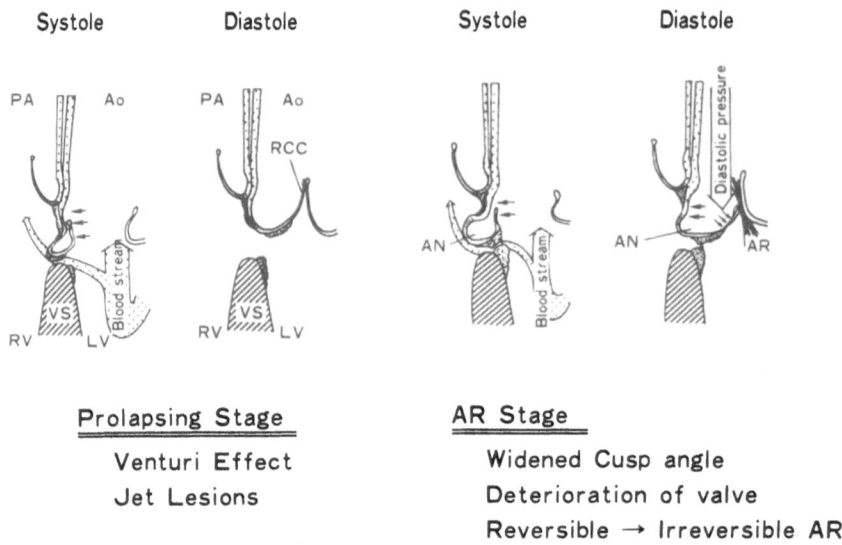

Systole   Diastole   Systole   Diastole

Prolapsing Stage   AR Stage

Venturi Effect   Widened Cusp angle

Jet Lesions   Deterioration of valve

Reversible → Irreversible AR

Fig. 10. Pathogenetic mechanism of prolapsing AR. For explanation see text. *VS* ventricular septum, *AN* aneurysm. Other abbreviations are as in previous figures

observed as a protrusion of the denuded sinus of Valsalva wall and cusp [16]. During diastole, as it returns to a normal position of the aortic valve, no protrusion is seen. The seesaw movement of the denuded sinus of Valsalva and cusp is angiographically interpreted as resulting from the "Venturi effect."

In addition to this effect, the anatomically unsupported sinus of Valsalva wall is pushed toward the right in every systole by aortic pressure, and this may induce dilatation of the valve annulus. This is the "prolapsing stage," i.e., the prodrome of prolapsing AR. As the disease progresses, the aortic valve becomes incompetent due to elongation of the free margin of the prolapsed cusp. But the Venturi effect is still present, and AR is still minimal. We call this stage the "reversible AR stage" because in the majority of patients at this stage competence of the valve is restored by simple closure of the defect [5, 6, 16]. Once AR develops, the diastolic pressure pushes down the prolapsed cusp and widens the cusp angle, resulting in the progression of AR. Due to jet lesions, the prolapsed cusp adheres with fibrous tissue to the margin of the VSD. The aortic valve itself had deteriorated with severe fibrous thickening induced by the jets. This is the "irreversible AR stage," in which the Venturi effect no longer exists, and the protrusion is relatively fixed in systole and diastole. Patients with a portion of weak and thin tissue at the denuded sinus of Valsalva wall or at the root of the prolapsed cusp may develop a huge aneurysm of the sinus of Valsalva. The functioning VSD in these cases is usually slitlike or closed, and AR is usually less than moderate with a relatively well-maintained valve angle. However, the huge aneurysm frequently ruptures into RV.

Clinical Implications

Based upon these anatomical observations and the hypothesis drawn from them, patients with IVSD should be operated on at, or preferably before, the reversible AR stage.

Therefore, a patient with IVSD should be regularly followed up, at least every 6 months, to detect the early signs of the onset of the AR. The aortic valve should be examined by either two-dimensional echocardiography or cineaortography to detect the prolapsing aortic valve [16]. Early or prophylactic surgical intervention is recommended even in those patients with malalignment-type VSD who have a deformed aortic valve and/or sinus of Valsalva wall anomalies. Although in the majority of these patients, dysfunction of the aortic valve appears to be inevitable, removal of the Venturi effect on the malformed aortic cusp may delay the onset of AR. If AR develops after surgery, isolated AR may usually progress slowly without compromising the child's development. Surgery for AR can be deferred until adolescence or later.

Acknowledgements. This work was supported by a Grant-in-Aid for Co-operative Research of the Japanese Educational Ministry (no. 56370021). We express our appreciation to Miss Miyuki Kahn and Mr. Hitoshi Miyabe for their technical assistance in preparing the manuscript.

References

1. Tatsuno K, Ando M, Takao A, Hatsune K, Konno S (1975) Diagnostic importance of aortography in conal ventricular septal defect. Am Heart J 89: 171-177
2. Ando M, Takao A (1978-1979) Racial differences in the morphology of common cardiac anomalies. Bulletin of the Heart Institute Japan: 47-66
3. Van Praagh R, McNamara JJ (1968) Anatomic types of ventricular septal defect with aortic insufficiency. Am Heart J 75: 604-619
4. Nadas A, Thilenius OG, LaFarge CG, Hauck AJ (1964) Ventricular septal defect with aortic regurgitation; Medical and pathologic aspects. Circulation 29: 862-873
5. Tatsuno K, Konno S, Ando M, Sakakibara S (1973) Pathogenetic mechanisms of prolapsing aortic valve and aortic regurgitation associated with ventricular septal defect. Circulation 48: 1028-1037
6. Tatsuno K, Konno S, Sakakibara S (1973) Ventricular septal defect with aortic insufficiency; Angiographic aspects and a new classification. Am Heart J 85: 13-21
7. Sakakibara S, Konno S (1968) Congenital aneurysm of the sinus of Valsalva associated with ventricular septal defect. Am Heart J 75: 593-603
8. Gonzalez-Lavin L, Barratt-Boyes (1969) Surgical consideration in the treatment of ventricular septal defect associated with aortic valve incompetence. J Cardiovasc Surg 57: 422-430
9. Someville J, Brandao A, Ross DH (1970) Aortic regurgitation with ventricular septal defect, surgical management and clinical features. Circulation 41: 317-330
10. Keane JF, Plath WH, Nadas AS (1977) Ventricular septal defect with aortic regurgitation. Circulation 56: I-72-77
11. Soto B, Becker AE, Mouleart AJ, Lie JT, Anderson RH (1980) Classification of ventricular septal defect. Br Heart J 43: 332-343
12. Goor DA, Edwards JE, Lillehei CW (1970) The development of the interventricular septum of human heart; correlative morphogenetic study. Chest 58: 453-467
13. Selzer A, Laqueun GL (1951) The Eisenmenger complex and its relation to the uncomplicated defect of the ventricular septum; Review of thirty-five autopsied cases of Eisenmenger complex, including two new cases. Arch Intern Med 87: 218
14. Goor DA, Lillehei CW, Rees R, Edwards JE (1970) Isolated ventricular septal defect. Developmental bases for various types and presentations of classification. Chest 58: 468-482
15. Momma K, Toyama K, Takao A, Nakazawa M, Hirosawa K, Imai Y (1984) Natural history of subarterial infundibular VSD. Am Heart J 108: 1312-1317
16. Tatsuno K, Ando M, Takao A, Hatsune K, Konno S (1975) Diagnostic importance of aortography in conal ventricular septal defect. Am Heart J 89: 171-177
17. de la Cruz MV, Campillo-Sainz C, Munoz-Armas S (1966) Congenital heart defect in chick embryos subjected to temperature variations. Circ Res 18: 257-262

Natural history and noninvasive of diagnosis of subpulmonic ventricular septal defect

Atsuyoshi Takao, Kazuo Momma, Kan Tohyama, Yoko Sawada, and Kazuhiro Mori

Studies made on surgical as well as on autopsy cases of ventricular septal defect (VSD) at our Institute have indicated that after the (peri)membranous type of VSD, subpulmonic VSD (SPVSD; subarterial infundibular) is the most frequent type of VSD, in contrast to the frequency reported in the Caucasian series. The purpose of this presentation is to review the natural history of SPVSD based on cases experienced at the Heart Institute, Tokyo Women's Medical College, and to discuss the specific features of various noninvasive diagnostic procedures identifying the subpulmonic location of VSD. The first part deals with the natural history. The natural history of SPVSD is unique in the following three aspects [1-3]: First, the aortic valve may prolapse into the SPVSD, resulting in aortic regurgitation [4-11]; second, aneurysm of the sinus of Valsalva may develop in association with the defect [11-13]; third, spontaneous closure rarely occurs.

Natural history of SPVSD

Understanding the natural history of SPVSD is necessary for better management of the condition. For this purpose, a total of 395 patients with SPVSD, all Japanese except for one Chinese and one Caucasian, 253 males and 142 females, who were admitted to the Heart Institute from 1972 through 1982, were studied. The study material discussed in the first part here is the same as that reported in Momma et al. [1].

Location of the VSD was confirmed at the time of intracardiac repair in 345 cases (87%) and diagnosed by left ventricular angiography in the other 50 cases (13%). Prolapse of the aortic cusp into the SPVSD was diagnosed either by retrograde aortography with aortic root injection in the lateral or right anterior oblique projection, or at the time of intracardiac repair. Aortic regurgitation was also diagnosed by aortography. Aneurysm of the sinus of Valsalva was diagnosed by aortography and open-heart surgery.

The age distribution of 95 patients with SPVSD, prolapse of the aortic valve, and aortic regurgitation (AR) is shown in Fig. 1. The youngest patients were 2 years old. In these two patients, a systolic murmur was present in infancy and an early diastolic decrescendo murmur appeared at 2 years of age. It can be seen that the peak age is 5-8 years. Most patients had been examined in our outpatient clinic twice yearly for a few years before cardiac catheterization. Some were studied by cardiac catheterization because of the appearance of a diastolic murmur. Others were studied with the tentative diagnosis of SPVSD and mild AR was first diagnosed by aortography.

Figure 2 illustrates the cumulative age distribution of 95 patients with SPVSD, prolapse of the aortic valve, and AR. Of the cases of prolapsing AR, 50% developed by the age of 8 years, and 87% by 20 years of age.

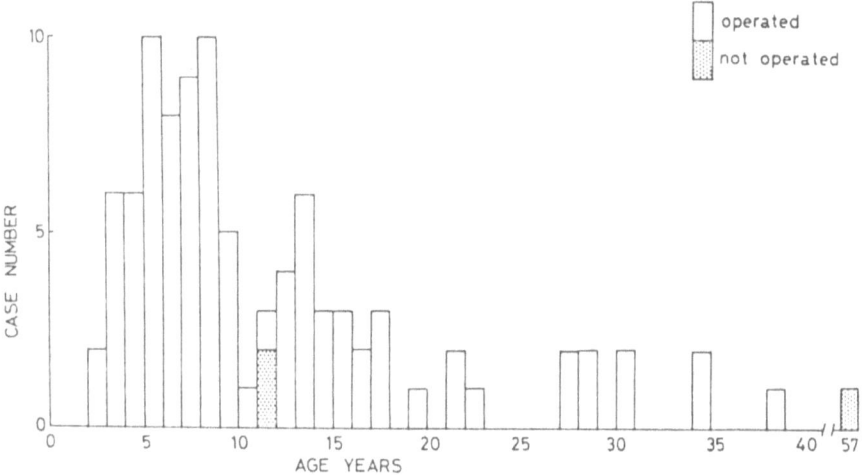

Fig. 1. Age distribution of 95 patients with SPVSD, prolapse of the aortic valve, and AR. (Reproduced from the Am. Heart J., vol. 108, p 1313 by permission)

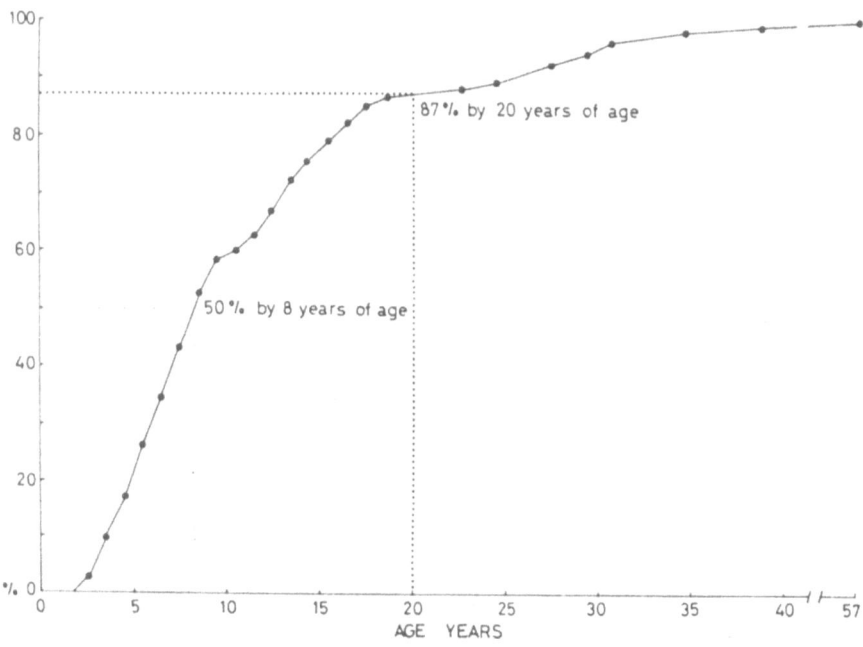

Fig. 2. Cumulative age distribution of patients with SPVSD, prolapse of the aortic valve, and AR. (Reproduced from the Am. Heart J., vol. 108, p 1314 by permission)

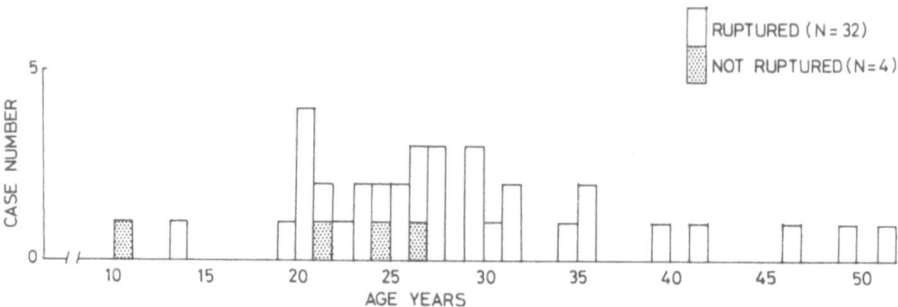

Fig. 3. Age distribution of 36 patients with SPVSD and aneurysm of the sinus of Valsalva. (Reproduced from the Am. Heart J., vol. 108, p 1315 by permission)

Figure 3 reveals the age distribution of 36 patients with SPVSD and aneurysm of the sinus of Valsalva. The aneurysm was ruptured in 32 cases but not in the remaining four cases. The youngest patient was 10 years old and only three cases were less than 20 years old. Rupture occurred most frequently in the third decade of life. Nonruptured aneurysm was diagnosed at a relatively young age (10–26 years). These cases were associated with variable degrees of AR.

Figure 4 shows the frequencies of complications of SPVSD in the eight age-groups. In 77 patients, aortic valvular prolapse without AR was noticed on aortography and the age distribution is shown here. VSD closure was done in all patients except one. These patients were mainly between 5 and 15 years of age, and were studied invasively because the findings of noninvasive diagnosis indicated a subpulmonic location of the VSD. Figure 4 shows that in each age-group the proportion of those patients with associated prolapse of the aortic valve gradually increased from 1% under 1 year of age to 70% at 15 years of age. In 76 patients, SPVSD was present and without prolapse, AR, or pulmonary hypertension (group 1). In 30 of 76 patients, the VSD was closed surgically and the absence of prolapse was confirmed. The proportion of these patients in each age-group decreased steadily from 5 to 7 years and no patient of this group was found after 31 years of age.

Thus, the natural history of SPVSD indicates the necessity for each detection of its localization of the VSD prior to the development of its complications and early assessment of the complications when they exist.

Figure 5 reveals the age distribution of each group of patients and shows that those having hyperkinetic hypertension with increased left-to-right shunt were mostly under 4 years of age. This group underwent an invasive study for definite surgical indication, although there were no signs of aortic valve prolapse or AR.

Noninvasive diagnosis of SPVSD

For this purpose, 89 consecutive cases of SPVSD (50 males and 39 females, 72 operated and 17 not operated) admitted to the Heart Institute from 1979 through 1983 were studied as to specific features of various noninvasive diagnostic findings obtained by physical examination, phonocardiogram, ECG, echocardiogram, and chest X-ray. The patients were pathophysiologically classified into five groups, i.e., simple subpulmonic

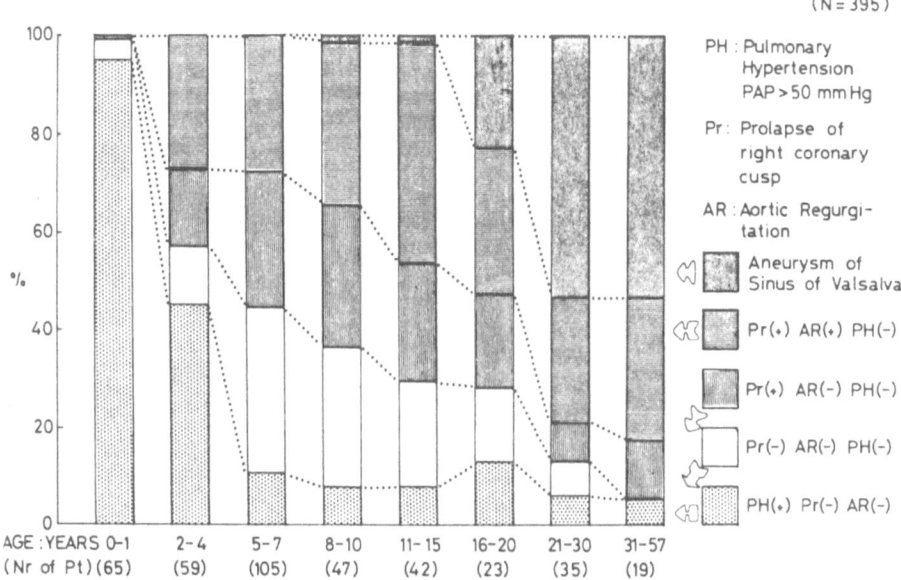

Fig. 4. Frequencies of complications of SPVSD in eight age-groups. The numbers of patients in each age-group are shown in *parentheses*. (Reproduced from the Am. Heart J., vol. 108, p 1315 by permission)

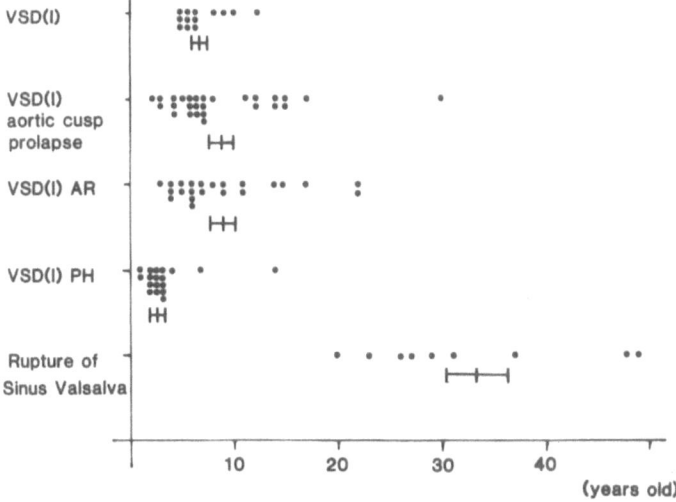

Fig. 5. Age distribution of 89 patients with SPVSD classified into five groups with or without complications. *VSD* (I) SPVSD

	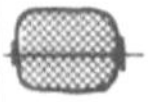 ⬭	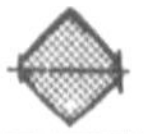 ◇	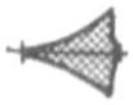 ◁	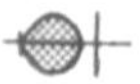 ⊙⊦	to and fro	SM DM
VSD(I)	6	2	5	0	0	0
VSD(I) aortic cusp prolapse	17	0	10	0	0	0
VSD(I) AR	8	0	6	0	0	7
VSD(I) PH	2	1	0	14	0	0
Rupture of Sinus Valsalva	0	0	0	0	9	0

Fig. 6. Patterns and characteristics of the phonocardiographic and auscultatory findings in each group of SPVSD.

(subarterial infundibular) VSD, those with aortic cusp prolapse, AR, pulmonary hypertension (PH), and ruptured sinus of Valsalva.

The physical findings of this group were those of hyperkinetic PH with increased pulmonary flow, consisting of overaccentuation of the pulmonic second sound with systolic murmur (mostly ejection in type), which was maximal at the second or third intercostal space, apical mitral flow murmur (or accentuated third heart sound), ECG evidence of biventricular hypertrophy, and cardiomegaly with increased lung vascularity in the chest X-ray. (However, this group did not have aortic valve prolapse or AR.) Except for this group, the most specific and diagnostic features were those of auscultatory findings and echocardiography, which detects the subpulmonic location of VSD and its complications or sequelae.

In 88 cases where phonocardiograms were available, 74 (84%) showed maximal intensity of the heart murmur located at the third to second intercostal space (ICS), and in the rest the murmur was heard maximally at the fourth ICS. The latter 14 cases included one with right coronary cusp (RCC) prolapse, two with prolapse and AR, five with ruptured sinus of Valsalva and AR, and six with hyperkinetic PH. Thus, in the majority of cases, the maximal intensity of the murmur of the SPVSD was located at the third to second ICS.

The pattern of the heart murmur was then analyzed according to each pathophysiological group (Fig. 6). In 57 cases of SPVSD, excluding those with definite (grade II–III) AR, ruptured sinus of Valsalva, or PH, the patterns of the heart murmur were classified into three types, i.e., band form in 31/54 (57%), diamond shape in 2/54 (4.3%), and crescendo late systolic accentuation type in 21/54 (38.7%). It is noteworthy that of 21 with the latter type, 16 (76%) revealed prolapse of the RCC. Those cases having definite AR (six) or ruptured sinus of Valsalva (nine) showed a biphasic murmur and to-and-fro murmur, respectively. The group with PH (15 cases) revealed auscultatory findings reflecting hyperkinetic hemodynamic findings according to the case, as mentioned before.

Electrocardiographically, in 58 cases, excluding those with definite AR, ruptured sinus of Valsalva (RSV), or PH, having a left-to-right shunt of less than 50% (55/58), the mean QRS axis of the frontal plane ranged from +30° to +90° in the majority of cases (Fig.

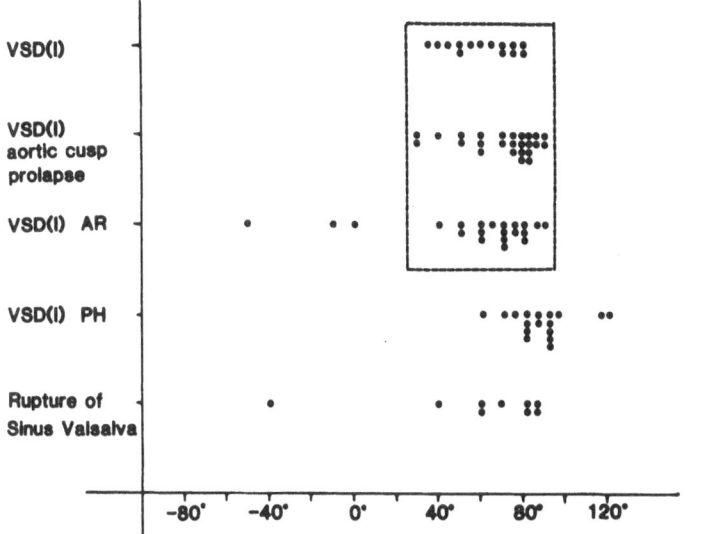

VSD(I)

VSD(I)
aortic cusp
prolapse

VSD(I) AR

VSD(I) PH

Rupture of
Sinus Valsalva

-80°   -40°   0°   40°   80°   120°

Fig.   7. Electrocar-
diographic   findings
in SPVSD

Table 1. Patients with surgically confirmed SPVSD categorized pathophysiologically and by age (n = 72)

Group	Diagnosis	Age range	mean	M-mode	2-DE
I	SPVSD + PH	5 mo – 7 yr,	1.6 yr	14	12
II	SPVSD	4 yr – 12 yr,	6.8 yr	14	10
III	SPVSD + RCC prolapse	3 yr – 30 yr,	8.7 yr	20	17
IV	SPVSD + RCC prolapse + AR	3 yr – 31 yr,	11.1 yr	17	17
V	SPVSD + RSV	20 yr – 56 yr,	34.9 yr	6	7

7). Marked left axis deviation was a rarity (3/58). In the horizontal plane, normal, left ventricular, or combined ventricular hypertrophic changes were observed, depending on the hemodynamic status of each individual case. No specific findings were seen in the chest X-ray; they only reflected the shunt status and pulmonary artery pressure.

Echocardiographic diagnostic features of SPVSD

The study material consisted of 72 consecutive patients with SPVSD whose diagnoses were confirmed at surgery. The age ranged from 5 months to 56 years. The patients were classified into five groups as follows (Table 1): Group I, SPVSD with PH; group II, SPVSD without PH and prolapse of the RCC; group III, SPVSD with prolapse of the RCC; group IV, SPVSD with prolapse of the RCC and AR; group V, SPVSD with RSV. M-mode echocardiography was done for 71 patients and two-dimensional echocardiography (2-DE) for 63 patients.

In the M-mode echocardiogram, as shown in Fig. 8, the distance from the anterior to the posterior wall of the sinus of Valsalva at end systole was designated as "a," the distance from the anterior wall of the sinus of Valsalva to the RCC was designated as "b," and the b/a ratio was then calculated. In 2-DE, the three indices of d/c, f/e, and h/g + h

M—mode

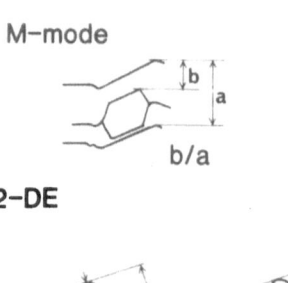

b/a

2-DE

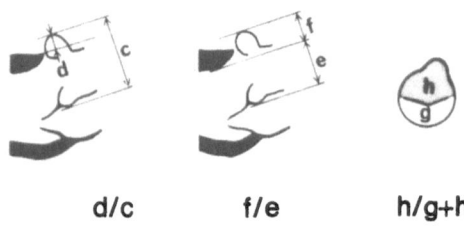

d/c   f/e   h/g+h

Fig. 8. Echocardiographic methods showing deformity of the aortic cusp and sinus of Valsalva using M-mode and 2-DE measurements

were determined to evaluate prolapse of the RCC as follows. In a long-axis view of the left ventricle, the largest diameter of the sinus of Valsalva was designated as "c," the distance from the anterior wall of the RCC to the right side of the inter-ventricular septum (IVS) was designated as "d," and the d/c ratio was obtained. The second index of the 2-DE was also calculated in the long-axis view of the left ventricle. The distance from the anterior wall of the RCC to the left side of the IVS was designated as "f," the distance from the left side of the IVS to the posterior wall of the sinus of Valsalva was designated as "e", and the f/e ratio was calculated. The third index using 2-DE was measured from the short-axis view of the aorta at the level of the aortic cusps. In the end-diastolic image of this view, the area of the RCC "h" and the whole area of the sinus of Valsalva "g + h" were measured, and the h/g + h ratio was computed.

Although the M-mode echocardiographic b/a ratio showed no significant differences among the five groups, there were some patients who showed very high values of the b/a ratio in groups III, IV, and V, but none in groups I and II (Fig. 9).

In Fig. 10, the 2-DE d/c ratios are shown. Relatively high values can be seen in groups III, IV, and V compared with groups I and II. The values of this index in patients with prolapse (groups III, IV, V) were significantly higher than in the nonprolapse groups (I, II).

In Fig. 11, the cases diagnosed by 2-DE as having prolapse of the RCC are shown by closed circles. When the value of this index was above 0.2, we were usually able to make a correct diagnosis of prolapsing RCC. (Existence of the RCC prolapse was proved by aortography or surgery.)

In Fig. 12, 2-DE f/e ratios are shown. These show a tendency to have higher values in the prolapsing groups (III, IV, V) than in the nonprolapsing groups (I, II).

In Fig. 13, the cases that were echocardiographically diagnosed as having prolapse of the RCC are shown by closed circles. When this index was above 1.0, our recognition of the prolapsing RCC was shown to be correct by a later invasive study or surgery. The percentage area of the RCC against the whole area of the sinus of Valsalva is shown in Fig. 14. There were no significant differences between the groups, but the cases with values above 0.5 were all in the prolapsing groups (III, IV, V).

In Fig. 15, the patients who were echocardiographically diagnosed as having prolapse

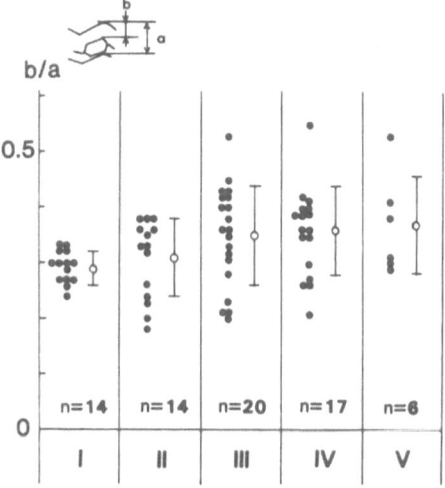

Fig. 9. M-mode b/a ratio among the five groups

of the RCC are shown by closed circles. When the value of h/g + h was above 0.5, our recognition of the RCC prolapse was correct. M-mode echocardiographic findings concerning fluttering of the pulmonary and mitral valves as well as aortic valve semiclosure were also studied (Table 2).

There was a significantly high ratio of pulmonary valve fluttering in SPVSD with PH (group I). Also, there was a significantly higher ratio of aortic valve semiclosure in the prolapsing groups (III), IV, V) than in the nonprolapsing groups (I, II).

The mitral valve fluttering was detected only in the two groups (IV, V) having AR. High detectability of RCC prolapse by 2-DE is expressed by high sensitivity (67%) and specificity (100%; Table 3).

Table 2. Fluttering of the pulmonary and mitral valves or aortic semiclosure among the five groups by M-mode echocardiography

	Group				
	I	II	III	IV	V
Pulmonary valve flutter (%)	94	44	55	28	67
Aortic valve semiclosure (%)	6	6	28	39	57
M-valve flutter (%)	0	0	0	33	33

Table 3. Detectability of RCC prolapse by 2-DE, showing high sensitivity (67%) and specificity (100%)

		2-DE	
		Positive (%)	Negative (%)
OP:	Positive (%)	19	9
	Negative (%)	0	24

Results shown for 52 patients. *OP*, confirmation of RCC prolapse by operation

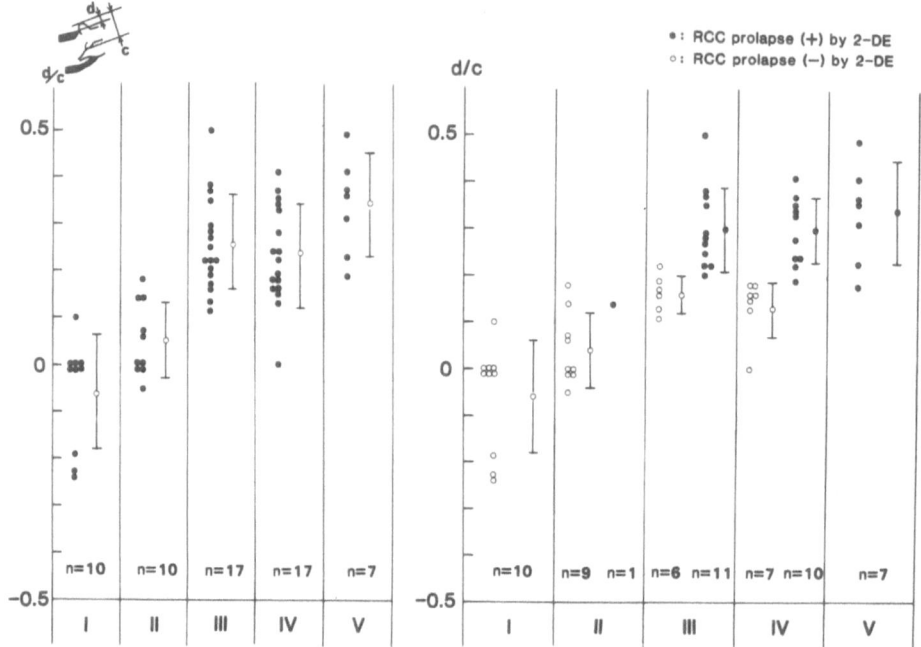

Fig. 10   Fig. 11

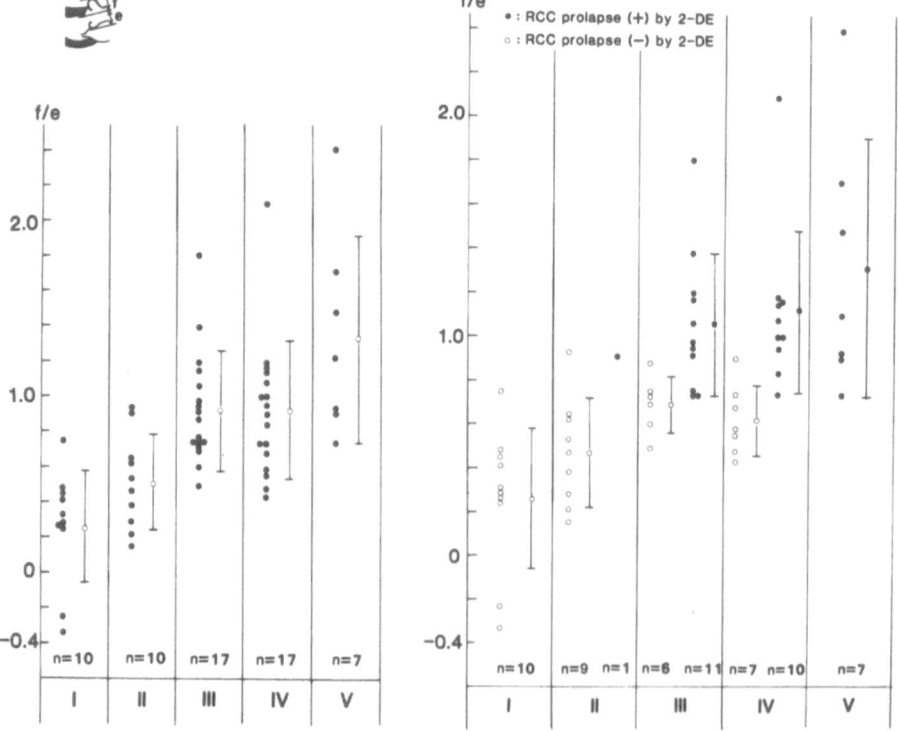

Fig. 12   Fig. 13

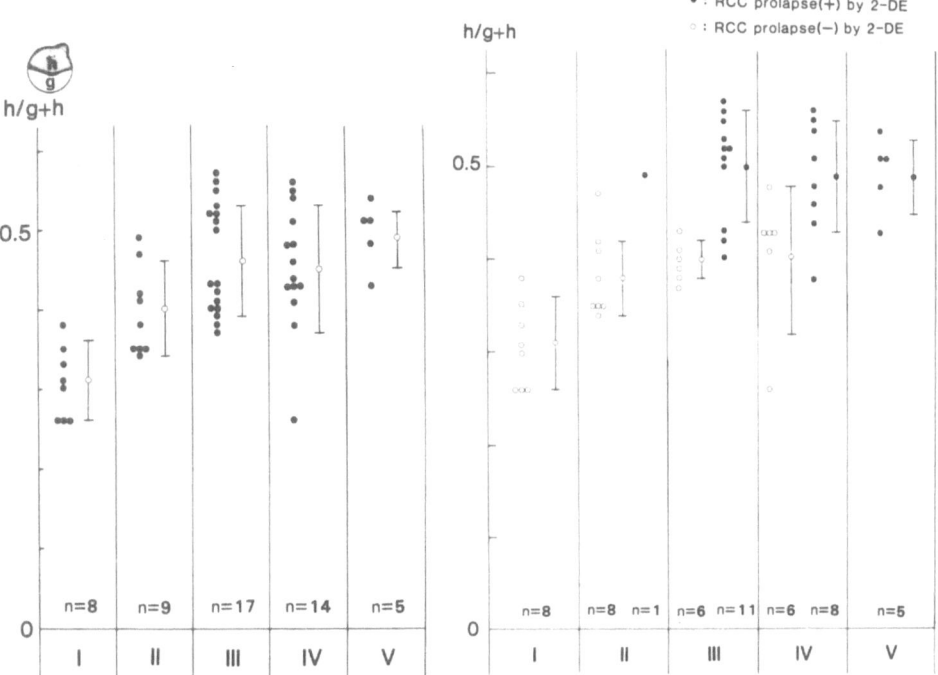

Fig. 14

Fig. 15

Fig. 10. 2-DE d/c ratio among the five groups indicating this value is significantly higher in the prolapse groups (III, IV, V) than in the nonprolapse groups (I, II)

Fig. 11. 2-DE d/c ratio among the five groups. Values above 0.2 indicate RCC prolapse

Fig. 12. 2-DE f/e ratio among the five groups showing a tendency of higher values in the prolapsing groups (III, IV, V)

Fig. 13. Values of 2-DE f/e ratio above 1.0 indicate higher recognition of RCC prolapse, which was later confirmed by an invasive study or surgery

Fig. 14. The percentage area of the RCC against the whole area of the sinus of Valsalva reveals no significant difference between the groups, but those with values above 0.5 were all in the prolapsing groups (III, IV, V)

Fig. 15. Values of h/g + h above 0.5 indicate correct recognition of RCC prolapse

Conclusion

Three hundred and ninety-five cases of SPVSD were studied to elucidate its natural history and the specific findings of various noninvasive diagnostic procedures. The natural history indicated the following: (1) With aging, SPVSD leads to prolapse of the right aortic cusp and then to AR, or to aneurysm of the sinus of Valsalva with or without regurgitation. (2) The cumulative age distribution of AR with SPVSD shows an appearance rate of AR of 50% by the age of 8 years and 87% by the age of 20 years, with the youngest patient being 2 years old. (3) Aneurysm of the sinus of Valsalva begins to appear during the third and fourth decades of life. Therefore, in order to prevent these complications, early detection and evaluation of aortic cusp prolapse or AR are imperative. Noninvasive diagnostic features indicative of SPVSD are as follows: (1) Localization of a systolic murmur maximal at the second and third ICS of the left sternal border and late systolic accentuation, suggestive of prolapse. (2) 2-DE evidence of right aortic cusp prolapse with pulmonary valve flutter or early semiclosure of the aortic valve. (3) Values obtained from the proposed indices of 2-DE showing high sensitivity and specificity for detecting the aortic cusp prolapse. (4) Mean frontal QRS $\hat{A}$ of $+30° - +90°$ in cases without PH, prolapse, or AR.

References

1. Momma k, Toyama K, Takao A, Ando M, Nakazawa M, Hirosawa K, Iami Y (1984) Natural history of subarterial infundibular ventricular septal defect. Am Heart J 108: 1312
2. Becker AE, Anderson RH (1981) Pathology of congenital heart disease. Butterworth & Co, Ltd., London, p 93
3. Soto B, Becker AE, Mouleart AJ, Lie JT, Anderson RH (1980) Classification of ventricular septal defect. Br Heart J 43: 332
4. Chung KJ, Manning JA (1974) Ventricular septal defect associated with aortic insufficiency: Medical and surgical management. Am Heart J 87: 435
5. Dimich I, Steinfeld L, Litwak RS, Park S, Silvers N (1973) Subpulmonic ventricular septal defect associated with aortic insufficiency. Am J Cardiol 32: 325
6. Goor DA, Lillehei CW (1975) Congenital malformations of the heart. Grune & Stratton, New York, p 297
7. Halloran KH, Talner NS, Browne MJ (1965) A study of ventricular septal defect associated with aortic insufficiency. Am Heart J 69: 320
8. Karpovich PP, Duff DF, Mullins CE, Cooley DA, McNamara DG (1981) Ventricular septal defect with associated aortic valve insufficiency. J Thorac Cardiovasc Surg 82: 182
9. Sakakibara S, Konno S (1968) Congenital aneurysm of the sinus of Valsalva associated with ventricular septal defect. Am Heart J 75: 595
10. Somverville J, Brandao A, Ross DN (1970) Aortic regurgitation with ventricular septal defect. Circulation 41: 317
11. Tatsuno K, Ando M, Takao A, Hatsune K, Konno S (1975) Diagnostic importance of aortography in conal ventricular septal defect. Am Heart J 89: 171
12. Plauth WH Jr, Braunwald E, Rockoff SD, Mason DT, Morrow AG (1965) Ventricular septal defect and aortic regurgitation: Clinical, hemodynamic and surgical considerations. Am J Med 39: 552
13. Sakakibara S, Konno S (1962) Congenital aneurysm of the sinus of Valsalva: Anatomy and classification. Am Heart J 63: 405

Global views:
State-of-the-art of ventricular septal defect
and coronary cusp prolapse

Ventricular septal defect with aortic regurgitation: Experience at a Korean center

C.Y. Hong, Y.S. Yun, J.Y. Choi, H.J. Kim, and Y.K. Lee

This study concerns patients with ventricular septal defect (VSD) with aortic regurgitation (AR) who underwent cardiac surgery at the Seoul National University Hospital, Seoul, Korea. During a period of 9 years from 1974 to 1982, a total of 2327 patients underwent open heart surgery (OHS). Among them, there were 1641 cases of congenital heart disease (CHD), and VSD comprised 39.4% of the total number of cases of operated CHD. There were 182 (28.2%) cases of subpulmonary VSD among the total 646 cases of VSD (Table 1).

Table 1. Annual number of cases of subpulmonic VSD

Year	OHS	CHD	VSD	Subpulmonic VSD	Percentage of subpulmonic VSD among VSD cases
1974	59	49	14	5	35.7
1975	53	39	10	5	50.0
1976	54	39	14	2	14.3
1977	100	65	18	6	33.3
1978	206	130	36	16	44.4
1979	320	220	65	17	26.2
1980	519	365	161	40	24.8
1982	600	446	215	63	29.3
Total	2327	1641	646	182	28.2

Of the total of 646 cases of VSD, subpulmonic VSD occured in 182 cases (28.2%), membranous defect in 384 (59.4%), AV canal defect in 69 (10.7%), muscular defect in five cases (0.8%), and combined defect (membranous and muscular) in six cases (0.9%), as shown in Table 2 and Fig. 1.

Table 2. Relative frequency of VSD type

Type	No. of cases	Percentage
Subpulmonic	182	28.2
Membranous	384	59.4
AV canal	69	10.7
Muscular	5	0.8
Combined	6	0.9
Total	646	100.0

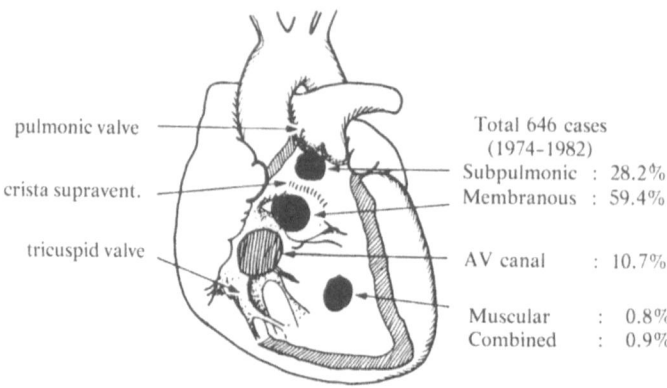

Fig. 1. Anatomic types of VSD

The age and sex distribution of VSD are show in Table 3. The male to female ratio was 1.7:1. There was no significant increase in the male/female ratio with age. Children less than 10 years of age comprised 72.8% of all VSD patients operated.

Table 3. Age and distribution of VSD

Age [years]	Sex		Male-Female ratio	Total
	Male	Female		
0–9	300	170	1.8	470
10–19	72	53	1.4	125
20–29	28	18	1.6	46
30–39	4			4
40–49	1			1
Total	405	241	1.7	646

Table 4 shows the relationship between age and type of VSD. In the first decade of life, 26.0% of cases of VSD were of the subpulmonic type; there were 34.4% in the second decade and 32.6% in the third decade and there was some tendency to increase with age, but this was not statistically significant ($P > 0.05$).

Table 4. Type of VSD by age-group

Age [years]	Subpulmonic type	Other types	Total
0–9	122 (26.0%)	348 (74.0%)	470
10–19	43 (34.4%)	82 (65.5%)	125
20–29	15 (32.6%)	31 (67.4%)	46
30–39	2 (50%)	2 (50%)	1
40–49		1	1
Total	182	464	646

The sex ratio in relation to age in VSD is shown in Table 5. There is a tendency for an increase in the male predominance with age in subpulmonic VSD ($P < 0.05$).

Table 5. Sex ratio (M/F) in relation to age and type of VSD

Age [years]	Subpulmonic type	Other types	Total
0-9	81/41 = 1.98	219/129 = 1.70	300/170 = 1.76
10-19	29/14 = 2.07	43/39 = 1.10	72/53 = 1.36
20-29	11/4 = 2.75	17/14 = 1.21	28/18 = 1.56
30-39	2/0	2/0	4/0
40-49		1/0	1/0
Total	123/59 = 2.08	282/182 = 1.55	405/241 = 1.68

The frequency of AR in various types of VSD is shown in Table 6. In subpulmonic VSD, 15.9% of the patients revealed AR, while in membranous VSD only 2.1% of the patients showed AR.

Table 6. Type of VSD with AR

Type	No. of cases	VSD + AR	Percentage
Subpulmonic	182	29	15.9
Membranous	384	8	2.1
AV canal	69	0	0
Muscular	5	0	0
Combined	6	0	0
Total	646	37	5.7

Of the 29 subpulmonic VSD patients with AR, 25 were males (M/F ratio = 6:1), while in membranous VSD with AR there was no sex difference (Table 7). Although there was a male preponderance even in subpulmonic VSD without AR (M/F ratio = 2:1), the difference was more prominent in cases with AR.

Table 7. Sex ratio (M/F) in VSD with AR

Age [years]	Subpulmonic VSD with AR	Membranous VSD with AR	Total
0-9	7/1	2/0	9/1
10-19	12/2	1/3	13/4
20-29	5/1	0/3	5/4
30-39	1/0		1/0
Total	25/4 (6:1)	3/5	28/9 (3:1)

The frequency of VSD with AR is shown by types of VSD and age-groups in Table 8. In each type, particularly in subpulmonic defects, the frequency of association with AR increases with age. The youngest patient was 4 years old. In subpulmonic VSD, 40% of the patients had associated AR in the third decade of life.

Table 8. VSD with AR by age-group

Age [years]	Total VSD	Subpulmonic VSD	Subpulmonic VSD with AR	Membranous VSD	Membranous VSD with AR
0–9	470	122	8 (6.6%)	292	2 (0.7%)
10–19	125	43	14 (32.6%)	68	3 (4.4%)
20–29	46	15	6 (40.0%)	22	3 (13.6%)
30–39	4	2	1	1	0
40–49	1	0	0	1	0
Total	646	182	29 (15.9%)	384	8 (2.1%)

Radiologically, most of the cases showed mild to moderate cardiomegaly with slightly increased pulmonary vascularity (Table 9). Aortography showed grade 2 or 3 aortic regurgitation in most cases.

Table 9. Radiological findings of VSD with AR

Cardiomegaly	−	+	+ +	+ + +	Total
Subpulmonic VSD with AR	3	9	11	6	29
Membranous VSD with AR	0	4	2	2	8
Total	3	13	13	8	37

The preoperative ECG findings are shown in Table 10. In most cases, the QRS axis was within normal limits and there was biventricular hypertrophy in 13.5% of cases.

Table 10. Preoperative ECG findings in VSD with AR

ECG findings		No. of cases	Percentage
QRS axis	Normal	34	91.9
	RAD	1	2.7
	LAD	2	5.4
Ventricular hypertrophy	No	4	10.8
	LVH	27	73.0
	BVH	5	13.5
	RVH	1	2.7

The cardiac catheterization findings are shown in Table 11. In 81% of the patients, the RV pressure was more than 30 mmHg. In about one-fourth of the patients, the pressure gradient between the RV and PA was more than 20 mmHg. In 62% of the cases, the QP/QS value was less than 2.

Congestive heart failure was observed in 19% (7/37) of the cases. There was evidence of bacterial endocarditis in 11% (4/37) of the cases.

Table 11. Cardiac catheterization findings

Catheterization finding		No. of cases	Percentage
RV pressure	< 30 mmHg	6	16.2
	30–60 mmHg	20	54.1
	≥ 60 mmHg	10	27.0
	Undetermined	1	
Pressure gradient	< 20 mmHg	26/34	76.5
RV→PA	≥ 20 mmHg	8/34	23.5
	< 1.5	12	32.4
QP/QS	1.5–2	11	29.7
	2–3	12	32.4
	≧3	2	5.4

The approximate size of the defects of the 37 patients is shown in Table 12. The size of the defects ranged from 0.5 to 3.5 cm, and in 65% (24/37) of the cases the defects were less than 2 cm in mean diameter.

Table 12. Size of VSD (mean diameter)

Size of defect	Subpulmonic type	Membranous type	Total
<0.6 cm	2		2
0.6–1.5 cm	12	5	17
1.5–2 cm	5		5
≥ 2 cm	10	3	13
Total	29	8	37

The method of operation in these 37 cases of VSD with AR is shown is Table 13. In 20 cases, only the VSD was closed, mostly by patch closure. In seven cases, valvuloplasty was performed in addition to the VSD closure. In ten cases, valve replacement was done. In this group,, the youngest patient was 10 years old.

Table 13. Operative method in VSD with AR

Method	Subpulmonic type	Membranous type
Direct suture	2	
Patch closure	13	5
Direct suture and valvuloplasty		1
Patch and valvuloplasty	6	
Direct suture and valve replacement	4	1
Patch and valve replacement	4	1
Total	29	8

There were four operative deaths out of 37 cases, and surgical fatality was 10.8%. Three deaths occurred in ten valve replacements, which was much higher than VSD without AR, in which surgical fatality was 2.0% (4/182) (Table 14).

Table 14. Operative fatality in VSD (1974-1982)

	Total VSD	Subpulmonic VSD
No. of cases	646	182
No. of operative deaths	26	4
Fatality rate [%]	4.0	2.2

The frequency of supracristal VSD in the present study is compared with that reported by other authors in Asian countries in Table 15.

Table 15. Frequency of subpulmonic VSD in Asian countries

Author Total no. VSD cases	Kawajima (174)	Tatsuno (93)	Chu (315)	Hong (646)
Subpulmonic	23	34.3	36.8	28.2
Membranous	77	63.4	61.3	59.4
AV canal	0	0	1.6	10.7
Muscular	0	2.2	0.3	0.8
Combined	0	0	0	0.9
Country	Japan	Japan	Taiwan	Korea
Year	1971	1971	1980	1983

Ventricular septal defect with aortic insufficiency in the Philippines

Wilberto L. Lopez

Ventricular septal defect (VSD) with aortic insufficiency (AI) has gained prominence as a syndrome as it almost invariably leads to diminished exercise tolerance and subsequent heart failure after a nonsymptomatic period ranging from 2 to several years. Nadas and his associates [1] reported an incidence of 4.6%, while Tatsuno et al [2] in 1973 quoted an incidence of 8.2%. Another important feature of the syndrome that the latter authors emphasized was the high incidence of subpulmonic VSD (78% of 91 cases). This is different from the incidence reported in the USA and Europe, where the subpulmonic and infracristal types of VSD occur with more or less equal frequency.

The object of this report is to determine the prevalence and incidence of VSD with complicating aortic insufficiency among Filipinos and to establish the type of VSD commonly involved in the syndrome.

Materials and methods

The 3415 patients who underwent hemodynamic studies at the Philippine Heart Center for Asia from April 1975 to October 1983 were reviewed. Table 1 shows a total of 456 cases of VSD, giving an incidence of 13.35%. Of these, isolated VSD accounted for 250 cases (54.8%), VSD with PS 95 cases (20.8%), VSD with ASD 28 cases (6.1%), VSD with PDA 31 cases (6.8%), VSD with AI 22 cases (4.8%), and VSD with other anomalies with normal vessels relationship 30 cases (6.6%). An analysis of the 22 cases of VSD with AI forms the basis of this report.

Table 1. Total number of VSD patients with cardiac catheterization (April 1975-October 1983)

	No. of patients
VSD isolated	250
VSD + PS	95
VSD + ASD	28
VSD + PDA	31
VSD + AI	22
VSD + other associated anomalies	30
Total	456

Total number of patients studied in the period was 3415

The classification of VSD with AI based on the location of VSD by Van Praagh and McNamara [3] was utilized in this paper.

Type I: infra- or subcristal VSD, which is located beneath the crista supraventricularis.

Type II: supracristal or subpulmonic VSD, which occurs below the pulmonic valve.

Type I was further subdivided into:

Type I-A: normal subpulmonic conus without infundibular stenosis.

Type I-B: some degree of underdevelopment of the subpulmonic infundibulum with a deviation of the supraventricularis away from the tricuspid valve to the anterior, superior, and left, giving rise to infundibular stenosis.

Results and discussion

Of the 22 cases reviewed, the age ranged from 2-17 years with a mean age of 9.5 years. There was a predominance of males over females (2:1 ratio; Fig. 1).

Table 2 shows the results of hemodynamic studies. Arterial oxygen saturation was normal in all except for case 22, in which arterial desaturation was caused by right-to-left shunt due to infundibular stenosis. A left-to-right shunt at the ventricular level was present in 21 patients with the Qp/Qs ratio ranging from 1.1:1 to 3.6:1. Wide pulse pressures were demonstrated in all with peak systolic pressures ranging from 90/30 (case 16) to 160/55 mm Hg (case 8).

Double step-ups in O_2 saturation were demonstrated in case 20 because of the presence of an associated PDA. Aortic stenosis was also noted in this case.

ECG and chest X-ray findings were reviewed and the cases were grouped into types I and II. Type I-A showed left ventricular hypertrophy (LVH) on ECG and type I-B had right ventricular hypertrophy (RVH). Cardiomegaly with left ventricular (LV) prominence in type I-A was seen on chest radiographs. In type I-B, one case had a normal-sized heart; cardiomegaly with right ventricular with (RV) prominence was seen in two cases. In type II, the ECG was normal in three cases; LVH in was noted in eleven cases, biventricular hypertrophy (BVH) in one. Chest X-rays showed a normal-sized heart in three cases. Cardiomegaly with LV prominence was seen in eight cases and it was biventricular in four (Table 3).

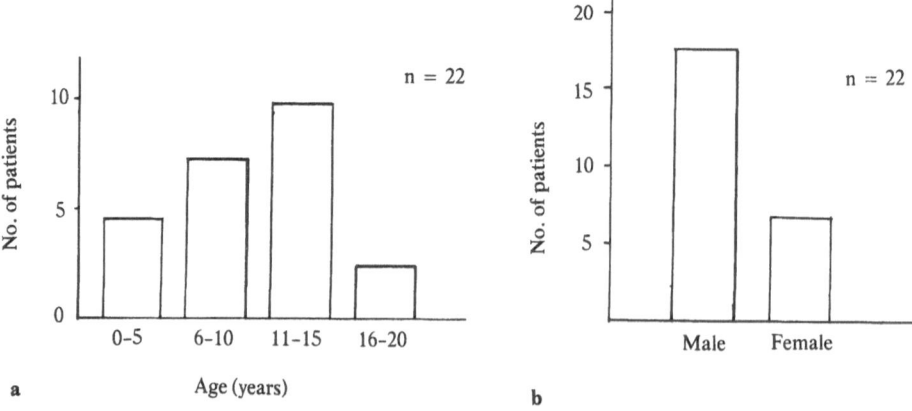

Fig. 1. a Age distribution of VSD with AI; **b** sex distribution of VSD with AI

Table 2. Cardiac catheterization data for VSD with AI ($n = 21$)

Case no.	Age [years]	Aorta O₂ Sat.	Aorta P		LV O₂ Sat. P	RV O₂ Sat. P	PA O₂ Sat.	PA P		Qp/Qs
1	11	95	$\frac{150}{85}$	110	96 $\frac{150}{10}$	85 $\frac{30}{7}$	83	$\frac{30}{10}$	20	1.5:1
2	7	91	$\frac{100}{30}$	55	90 $\frac{100}{10}$	83 $\frac{25}{6}$	82	$\frac{22}{6}$	14	1.7:1
3	14	97	105	65	95 $\frac{105}{10}$	83 $\frac{30}{5}$	83	$\frac{27}{10}$	15	1.2:1
4	8	92	$\frac{105}{45}$	65	92 $\frac{105}{15}$	78 $\frac{30}{5}$	78	$\frac{30}{17}$	18	1.3:1
5	12	94	$\frac{100}{66}$	90	94 $\frac{100}{10}$	85 $\frac{65}{10}$	85	$\frac{25}{10}$	15	2.0:1
6	15	94	$\frac{100}{50}$	80	94 $\frac{100}{10}$	83 $\frac{24}{12}$	84	$\frac{24}{12}$	15	1.2:1
7	17	91	$\frac{120}{30}$	65	90 $\frac{120}{10}$	80 $\frac{25}{4}$	81	$\frac{25}{10}$	13	1.1:1
8	10	91	$\frac{160}{55}$	100	91 $\frac{160}{15}$	81 $\frac{70}{10}$	83	$\frac{42}{24}$	30	1.6:1
9	4	91	$\frac{100}{50}$	70	90 $\frac{100}{10}$	80 $\frac{48}{5}$	79	$\frac{25}{8}$	15	1.8:1
10	14	92	$\frac{120}{65}$	80	93 $\frac{120}{20}$	77 $\frac{50}{5}$	83	$\frac{30}{13}$	17	1.2:1
11	11	—	$\frac{110}{65}$	85	93 $\frac{110}{10}$	83 $\frac{22}{5}$	84	$\frac{25}{13}$	18	1.5:1
13	2	92	$\frac{120}{55}$	80	91 $\frac{120}{15}$	79 $\frac{20}{5}$	79	$\frac{20}{12}$	14	1.7:1
14	9	95	$\frac{80}{35}$	60	94 $\frac{80}{10}$	75 $\frac{20}{5}$	76	$\frac{20}{5}$	10	1.2:1
15	17	93	$\frac{105}{60}$	75	93 $\frac{105}{5}$	80 $\frac{20}{6}$	81	$\frac{20}{8}$	14	1.6:1
16	3	96	$\frac{90}{30}$	60	95 $\frac{90}{15}$	87 $\frac{55}{10}$	86	$\frac{55}{20}$	35	3.6:1
17	10	95	$\frac{100}{44}$	64	95 $\frac{100}{12}$	90 $\frac{30}{4}$	89	$\frac{30}{10}$	17	2.1:1
18	14	95	$\frac{105}{40}$	75	95 $\frac{110}{5}$	83 $\frac{27}{2}$	84	$\frac{17}{8}$	12	1.3:1
19	3	92	$\frac{105}{55}$	75	92 $\frac{105}{5}$	86 $\frac{25}{3}$	84	$\frac{25}{12}$	18	1.9:1
20	8	95	$\frac{105}{50}$	80	98 $\frac{130}{10}$	80 $\frac{120}{10}$	88	$\frac{100}{30}$	55	2:1
21	14	96	$\frac{90}{38}$		96 $\frac{90}{8}$	92 $\frac{40}{4}$	92	$\frac{30}{10}$		3.6:1
22	14	85	$\frac{100}{75}$	80	89	70	No pressure taken			—

Case 12 did not undergo hemodynamic study, O_2 Sat. oxygen saturation, P pulse pressure

Table 3. ECG and chest radiographic findings in VSD with AI ($n = 21$)

Type of VSD with AI (no. of cases)	Electrocardiographic findings (no. of cases)	Chest radiographs (no. of cases)
Type I-A (2)	LVH (1) LVH (1)	Cardiomegaly, LV prominence (2)
Type I-B (4)	RVH (4)	Normal-sized heart (1) Cardiomegaly, RV prominence (3)
Type II (15)	WNL (3) LVH (11) BVH (1)	Normal-sized heart (3) Cardiomegaly with LV prominence (8) Cardiomegaly with biventricular prominence (4)

Table 4. Aortic valve leaflet involvement in VSD with AI, type I ($n = 6/22$)

Subtype	Case no.	Age [years]/ sex	Aortic valve (Angiographic)		Pulmonary gradient	Management	
			Leaflet prolapse	Aortic regurgitation		Medical	Surgical
I-A	11	11/M	NCC	4+	(−)		VSD closure AVR
I-A	21	14/M	RCC	4+	10-mmHg		VSD closure AVR
I-B	5	12/F	RCC	3+	40-mmHg	(+)	
I-B	9	4/F	RCC[a]	2+	23-mmHg		VSD closure
I-B	20	8/M	RCC	1+	20-mmHg	(+)	
I-B	22	14/M	RCC	3+	RV = 125/20		VSD closure Rastelli external conduit

NCC noncoronary cusp, *RCC* right coronary cusp, *AVR* aortic valve replacement
[a] Both NCC and RCC were found prolapsed at surgery

Analysis of the type of VSD and aortic valve leaflet involvement was done and the data are summarized in Table 4. Type I-A involved the noncoronary cusp. Type I-B with associated infundibular stenosis involved mainly the right coronary cusp. Four patients underwent surgery with patch closure of the VSD and in addition two patients had aortic valve replacement and another (case 22) had a Rastelli external conduit. Two other patients refused surgery.

Type II numbered 15 cases in all (Table 5). The right coronary cusp was involved in all except for cases 3 and 6 in which the noncoronary cusp of the aortic valve was involved. Case 8 had prolapse of both the right and noncoronary cusps.

Eight of the fifteen patients underwent VSD patch closure plus valvuloplasty in four and aortic valve replacement in three patients. One patient underwent VSD closure only. The rest elected to be treated medically.

Operative findings were checked and are listed in Table 6. All patients had 3+ to

Table 5. Aortic valve leaflet involvement in VSD with AI, type II ($n = 15/22$)

Case no.	Age [years]/ sex	Aortic valve		Pulmonary gradient [mmHg]	Management	
		Leaflet prolapse	Aortic regurgitation		Medical	Surgical
1	11/M	RCC	4+	(−)	(+)	
2	7/M	RCC	4+	(−)	(+)	
3	14/M	NCC	2+	(−)	(+)	
4	8/M	RCC	4+	(−)	(+)	
6	15/F	NCC	2+	(−)		VSD closure
7	17/M	RCC	4+	(−)		VSD closure AVR
8	10/M	RCC/NCC	4+	30		VSD closure AVR
10	14/M	RCC	3+	20		VSD closure AVR
13	2/M	RCC	2+	(−)	(+)	
14	9/M	RCC	3+	(−)	(+)	
15	17/F	RCC	2+	(−)		VSD closure, plication of aneurysm sinus of Valsalva
16	3/F	RCC	3+	(−)		VSD closure AVA
17	10/M	RCC	3+	(−)		VSD closure AVA
18	14/M	RCC	4+	10		VSD closure
19	3/M	RCC	2+	(+)		

AVR Aortic valve replacement, *AVA* aortic valve annuloplasty

Table 6. Operative findings in VSD with AI ($n = 12/21$)

Case no.	Age at operation [years]	Coronary cusp prolapse	AO valve repair	VSD pathology
6	15	NCC	(−)	Subpulmonic
7	17	RCC	AVR	Subpulmonic, 2.5 × 1.5 cm
8	10	NCC-RCC	AVR	Subpulmonic, 1.0 × 1.0 cm
9	4	NCC-RCC	(−)	Subcristal
10	14	RCC	AVR	Subpulmonic
11	11	RCC	AVR	Subpulmonic
15	17	NCC	Plication aneurysm of sinus of Valsalva	Subpulmonic
16	3	RCC	AO valve annuloplasty	Subpulmonic, 1.5 cm
17	10	RCC	AO valve annuloplasty	Subpulmonic, 1.5 cm
18	14	RCC	AVR	Subpulmonic
21	14	RCC	AVR	Subcristal
22	14	NCC	(−)	Subcristal

NCC Noncoronary cusp, *RCC* right coronary cusp, *AVR* aortic valve replacement, (−) surgery was not done on aortic valve

4 + AI on angiograms except for cases 6 and 9, who had 2 + AI and received only VSD patch closure. Cases 16 and 17 had 3 + AI and received valve annuloplasty in addition to closure of the VSD. The rest of the patients who had 4 + AI received aortic valve replacement in addition to VSD closure. Plication of the aneurysm of the sinus of Valsalva was done in case 15, and a Rastelli external conduit was performed in case 22. All patients survived and showed improvement.

Operative findings regarding the type of VSD and aortic cusp involved tallied with the angiocardiographic diagnosis except for case 9, in which both right and noncoronary cusps rather than the right cusp alone were found prolapsed at surgery.

In summary, VSD with AI occurred in 4.8% of 456 cases of VSD that underwent hemodynamic studies. In those cases complicated with AI, subpulmonic VSD (type II) comprised 68% of the cases studied. The right coronary cusp is the most common cusp to prolapse with occasional involvement of the noncoronary cusp. Subpulmonic VSD is relatively common among Filipinos. Surgery is recommended for VSD with complicating AI when clinical and hemodynamic indications are evident [4, 5].

References

1. Nadas AS Thilenius OG Lafarge CG, and Hauck AJ (1964) Ventricular septal defect with aortic regurgitation: Medical and pathologic aspects. Circulation 29: 862
2. Tatsuno K, Konno S, Sakakibara S (1973) Ventricular septal defect with aortic insufficiency: Angiocardiographic aspects and a new classification. Am Heart J 85: 13–21
3. Van Praagh R, McNamara JJ (1968) Anatomic types of ventricular septal defect with aortic insufficiency, Am Heart J 75: 604
4. Spencer FC, Bahnson HT Neil CA (1962) The treatment of aortic regurgitation associated with VSD. J Thorac Cardiovasc Surg 43: 222–233
5. Gonzalez-Lavin L, Barratt-Boyes BG (1969) Surgical consideration in the treatment of ventricular septal defect associated with aortic valvular incompetence. J Thorac Cardiovasc Surg 57: 422–430

Aortic regurgitation and aortic valve cusp deformity in ventricular septal defect in India

I.P. Sukumar, Y. Varma, and C. Babu Uthaman

A prospective study of 50 consecutive cases of ventricular septal defects (VSD) by aortic root cine angiocardiography in two projections is reported. Aortic valve cusp deformity (AVCD) was found in 43 cases (86%). The AVCD involved the non-coronary cusp (NCC) alone in 50%, right coronary cusp (RCC) and NCC in 14%, RCC alone in 18% and left coronary cusp (LCC) alone in 4% of cases. Relating AVCD to the type of VSD, four of five cases with supracristal VSD and 37 of 45 cases with infracristal VSD had AVCD. Aortic regurgitation (AR) was found in 34% of cases, as compared with 14.5% in an earlier retrospective study of 350 cases of VSD. AR was mild in 24%, moderate in 8% and severe in 2% of cases. The jet of AR was to the left ventricle (LV) alone in 22% and to both the right ventricle (RV) and LV in 12% of cases; the NCC was involved in ten (20%) and the NCC plus the RCC in four (8%), the RCC alone in two (4%) and the LCC alone in no patients. All patients except one with AR had AVCD. AR does not appear to influence the development of pulmonary hypertension, as 34 patients (68%) had normal pulmonary artery (PA) pressure, including one patient with severe AR. Two patients with AVCD without AR pre-operatively developed AR 6 months and 1 year after VSD closure and none had residual VSD.

It is postulated that AVCD and AR are more frequent in VSD in India than reported earlier. AVCD without AR is important as patients may subsequently develop AR even after VSD closure. VSD is a common congenital malformation seen either as an isolated anomaly or in combination with other congenital cardiac malformations. Association of AR in VSD has been a matter of interest in recent years as it alters the clinical and haemodynamic features and the resultant AR may lead to an additional burden on the LV. The incidence of AR in VSD reported from different parts of the world has varied from 0.6% to 5%. However, since a report from Japan showed an incidence of nearly 10% there has been the increasing belief that AR in VSD is more frequent in Asian countries. A prospective study of the incidence of AR and aortic cuspal deformities in isolated VSD in Indian patients was undertaken. A retrospective study from this centre showed an incidence of 14.5% out of 350 cases of VSD.

Fifty consecutive cases of isolated VSD were studied from 1982 to 1983 in our institution irrespective of patient age, symptoms or magnitude of shunts. Patients with a history suggestive of infective endocarditis or rheumatic fever and those with a bicuspid aortic valve were excluded from the study. The age ranged from 5 to 45 years with a mean of 16.2 years. The male to female ratio was 2.3:1. All had clinical evidence of VSD. Forty-five patients had infracristal and five supracristal VSD; there were no cases of muscular VSD. Five patients had a high-pitched decrescendo early diastolic murmur along the left sternal border, suggesting associated AR. In the remaining 12 patients, AR was diagnosed angiographically but could not be detected clinically. Aortic root cine angiograms in standard RAO and LAO views were used to define the cuspal anatomy and assess the presence and severity of AR. The severity of AR was assessed by modified Sellers' criteria [1] and was classified as mild, moderate or severe. Aortic valve cusp deformity was diagnosed when the cusp was seen to prolapse, sag or herniate in either or both ventricles or appear irregularly deformed.

Seventeen patients had a small left-to-right shunt with a Qp/Qs ratio of <1.5:1. Eighteen patients had flow ratios of between 1.5:1 and 2:1, fourteen had flow ratios of >2:1 and one had a bidirectional shunt. The pulmonary artery systolic pressure was normal at less than 35 mmHg in 34 patients. Only 12 patients had more than moderate pulmonary hypertension (pulmonary arterial pressure >50 mmHg). Of the 50 patients, 43 showed abnormalities of the valve cusp. The NCC alone was involved in twenty-five, the RCC alone in nine, both RCC and NCC in seven and deformity of the LCC was found in only two patients. Of the 50 patients, 17 (35%) had AR of varying severity. Twelve patients were classified as mild, four as moderate and one had severe AR. The regurgitant jet was to the LV alone in eleven and to both the RV and LV in six patients; there were no cases of the RV alone. The 12 patients with mild AR angiographically showed no clinical signs. Relating cuspal deformity with AR, the NCC alone was abnormal in ten cases (Fig. 1), NCC and RCC together in four cases (Fig. 2) and the RCC alone in two cases (Fig. 3). One patient had a normal cusp, none had an abnormal LCC. Two patients, one with supracristal and one with infracristal VSD, had an abnormal NCC and no AR pre-operatively (Fig. 1). Both developed AR 6 months and 12 months after closure of the VSD. There was no residual VSD in either of these patients.

Laubry and associates [5] in 1933 first recognized this combination in an 18-year-old boy and this was later confirmed at autopsy. Various reports have put the incidence between 3% and 5%, except in Japan where the incidence has been reported as 10%. Wood et al. [3] in 1954 reported two patients with this combination when they studied 60

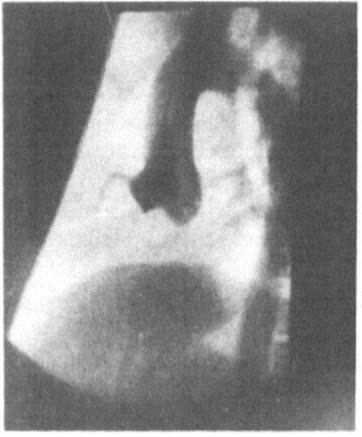 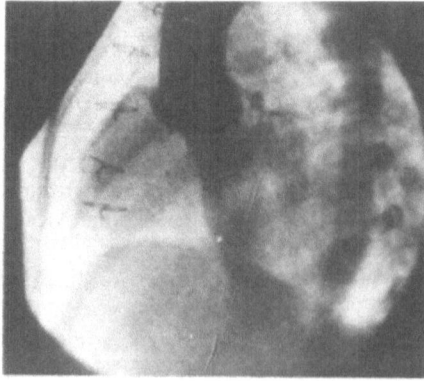

Fig. 1. Abnormal non-coronary cusp, no aortic regurgitation pre-operatively. Post-operative aortic root angiography shows aortic regurgitation

patients with isolated, uncomplicated VSD. Nadas et al. [2] found 34 of 756 patients with VSD had AR, an incidence of almost 5%. Plauth et al. [6] encountered an incidence of 6.6% of prolapse of an aortic leaflet leading to AR in VSD. Weidman et al. [4] reported an incidence of 0.6%.

Our study of 50 consecutive case of VSD reveals that the incidence of aortic cuspal abnormality and AR is much higher in India than in Western countries. The cause for this high incidence is not clear. Aortic cuspal abnormality was detected in 43 of the 50 patients (86%), involving the NCC in twenty-five (50%), RCC in nine (18%), both RCC

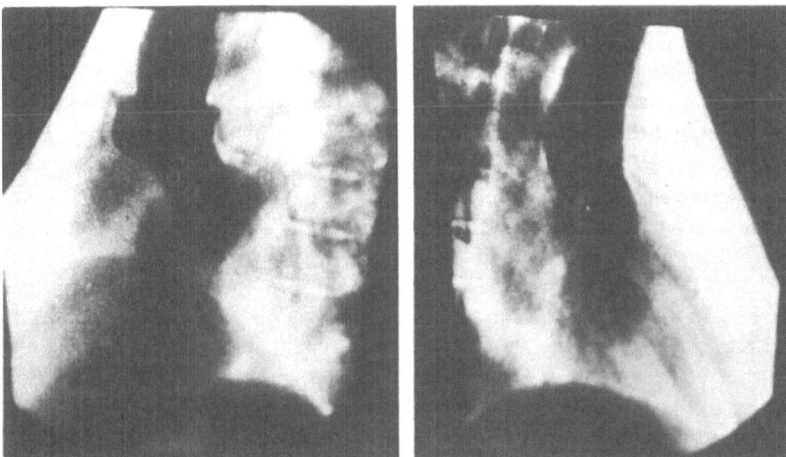

Fig. 2. Abnormal non-coronary and right coronary cusp with aortic regurgitation to right and left ventricle.

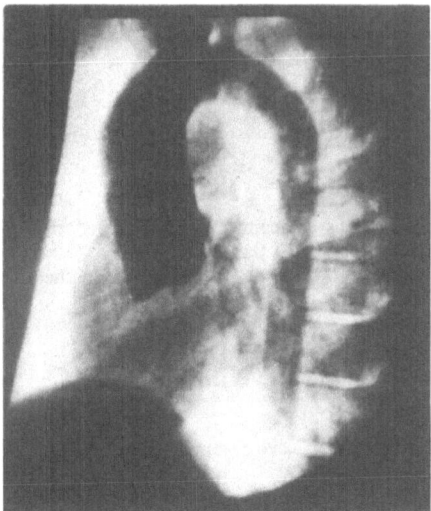

Fig. 3. Abnormal right coronary cusp. Aortic regurgitation to left ventricle

and NCC in seven (14%) and LCC in two (4%). Sixteen patients with cuspal abnormality had AR. Only one patient had AR with normal aortic valve cusps.

The ratio of males to females in the previously reported cases was 1.8:1 and of these, three-fourths were 15 years old or younger. Our study showed a male predominance, with a ratio of 2.3:1. Twenty-five patients (50%) were under 11 years of age and seven (14%) were between 20 and 45 years, thus indicating that AR can develop at any time if the aortic valve cuspal abnormality exists. The jet of AR to the LV alone was seen in eleven (22%) and to both LV and RV in six patients (12%).

The magnitude of the shunt does not appear to affect the development of AR as only 14 (28%) had a Qp/Qs ratio of more than 2:1; neither does the anatomical position of the VSD. The literature indicates a higher incidence of AR in supracristal VSD [4, 7, 8] but the phenomenon is by no means rare in infracristal VSD.

A previous reports indicated that the RCC was most commonly affected (75%) in the 68 patients for whom a specific anatomical description was given. The NCC cusp was pro-lapsed in seven (10%), both NCC and RCC in nine (13%) and LCC in one patient [10]. Our evidence shows that the most commonly deformed cusp was the NCC in 50%, RCC in 18%, both RCC and NCC in 14% and LCC in only two patients. Of the 25 cases with deformed NCC alone, ten had AR, and of the seven with deformed RCC and NCC, four had AR. The involvement of isolated RCC deformity with AR was only seen in two patients. No patients with deformed LCC alone had AR.

Spencer et al. [11] suggested that the usual mechanism of prolapse may be initial descent of the base of the unsupported aortic leaflet until the free edge of the leaflet lies at a level lower than that of the other leaflets. The regurgitant blood impinges upon the malpositioned free edge of the leaflet, which lengthens progressively. However, Dentsch et al. [12] attributed the development of AR to the abnormal position of the membranous septum, resulting in deficient support for the aortic valve cusps.

Neither of these hypotheses explain why there should be a higher incidence of aortic valve cusp deformity and AR in Indian and other Asian patients. However, in two cases where AR developed after closure of VSD, these hypotheses may not be applicable. A possible mechanism in these two cases could be that a prolapsing cusp due to abnormal position of membranous septum becomes weak and malaligned and this malalignment ultimately produces aortic insufficiency. It is postulated that aortic valve cusp deformity in VSD and AR is more frequent in India than has been reported for Western countries. AVCD without AR is important as patients with this condition may develop AR at a later stage even after a successful VSD closure.

References

1. Sellers RD, Lexy MJ, Amplatz K (1964) Left retrograde cardioangiography in acquired cardiac disease. Technic, indications and interpretations in 700 cases. Am J Cardiol 14: 437
2. Nadas AS, Thilenius OG, La Farge CG Hauck AJ (1964) VSD with AR: Medical and pathologic aspects. Circulation 29: 862–873
3. Wood P, Magidson O, Wilson PAO (1954) VSD with note on acyanotic Fallot's tetralogy. Br Heart J 16: 387–406
4. Weidman WH, Blount SG Jr, Dushane JW, Gensony WM, Mayes CJ, Nadas AS (1977) Clinical course of VSD. Circulation 56 (Suppl) 1
5. Laubry C, Routier D, Soutre P (1933) Les souffles de la maladie de Roger. Rev Med Interne 50: 439
6. Plauth WH, Braunwald E, Rockoff SD, Mason DT, Morrow AG (1965) Am J Med 39: 552–567
7. Edwards JE (1958) Pathologic aspects of cardiac valvular insufficiencies. Arch Surg 77: 634
8. Taussig MB, Semans JH (1940) Severe aortic insufficiency in association with a congenital malforma-tion of the heart of the Eisenmenger type. Bulletin of John Hopkins Hospital 66: 156

9. Kawashima Y, Danno M, Shimizu Y, Matsuda H, Myamoto T, Fugita T, Kozuka T, Manabe H (1973) VSD associated with AR, Anatomic classification and method of operation. Circulation 47: 1057
10. Starr A, Menashe V, Dotter C (1960) Surgical correction of aortic insufficiency associated with VSD. Surg Gynecol Chest 111: 71
11. Spencer FC, Bahson HT, Neill CA (1962) The treatment of AR associated with VSD. J Thorac Cardiovasc Surg 43: 222
12. Dentsch, Blieden LC, Krans Y, Yahini JH (1969) VSD associated with AR. Am J Roentgen Radiother 106

Ventricular septal defect and coronary cusp prolapse: Experience at a European center

Lucas G. Van der Hauwaert, Monique Dumoulin, Willem Daenen, and Georges Stalpaert

Between January 1973 and June 1983, 220 consecutive patients, aged 2 months to 40 years, underwent surgical closure of an uncomplicated ventricular septal defect (VSD). All patients had undergone preoperative cardiac catheterization. Patients with tetralogy of Fallot, atrioventricular septal defect, and transposition or malposition of the great arteries were excluded. Also excluded were patients with associated coarctation or valvular anomalies, except aortic insufficiency.

The anatomical locations of the VSD, identified at surgery, were as follows: perimembranous 167 (76%), supracristal 13 (6%), right ventricular inlet type 10 (4.5%), muscular 9 (4%), atrioventricular canal type 1, combination of a perimembranous defect with another type 4, undetermined 15. In 19 of 220 patients (8.6%), aortic insufficiency (AI) was diagnosed preoperatively and confirmed at operation (Table 1). AI was a complication in 13 of 167 cases of perimembranous VSD (7.8%) and 6 of 13 cases of supracristal VSD (46%).

The anatomical substrate of the AI in 13 patients with a perimembranous VSD was variable: prolapse of the right coronary cusp (RCC) in five patients, prolapse of the non-coronary cusp (NCC) in four, aneurysm of the NCC in one, prolapse of both the RCC and NCC with a hypoplastic left coronary cusp (LCC) in one, severe retraction of the NCC in one, and prolapse of the RCC with calcification of the commissure between the RCC and NCC in one. In four of the six patients with a supracristal VSD and associated AI, the AI was caused by prolapse of the RCC; in one patient it was caused by prolapse of the NCC and its commissure with the RCC, and in the remaining patient by prolapse and fenestration of both the RCC and LCC. Protrusion of an aortic cusp into the VSD was noticed in only three of the nineteen patients with aortic insufficiency — two had a supracristal VSD and one a perimembranous VSD.

Table 1. Incidence of associated aortic insufficiency

Site of VSD	No. of patients	No. with AI
Perimembranous	167	13 (7.8%)
Supracristal	13	6 (46%)
Other types	40	0
All types of VSD	220	19 (8.6%)

At the time of operation, 14 of the 19 patients were under 10 years of age; the mean age was 9.5 years. The VSD was closed by patch insertion in twelve patients and by direct suturing in seven. Efforts were always made to preserve the aortic valve. In 17 of 19 patients, a valvuloplasty was performed. It basically consisted of shortening the free margin of the elongated cusp and suturing widened or prolapsing commissures. In the two oldest patients, aged 18 and 37 years, a severely deformed valve had to be excised and was replaced by a mechanical device. There was no hospital or late mortality. In four patients only was the AI abolished by valvuloplasty. A reduction of the aortic leak was achieved in 11 cases. However, 2 of these 11 patients required reoperation and valve replacement because of persisting severe AI: In one patient this was peformed 2 weeks after the first operation and in the other patient after 7 years. At the last follow-up examination, all 19 patients were asymptomatic and leading a normal life. The VSD had remained closed in all. The four patients who underwent aortic valve replacement had no complications from this procedure. Of the 15 patients who had undergone aortic valvuloplasty, four had a competent aortic valve, and 11 a slight or moderate degree of aortic regurgitation.

Conclusions

Supracristal or subpulmonic VSD is rare in the European population (6% in the present series) and its incidence is far below that found in some Asian, particularly Japanese, series. Approximately 9% of 220 consecutive, otherwise uncomplicated cases of VSD were associated with AI. In these patients, a perimembranous VSD was twice as common as a supracristal VSD, which is also in contrast to the figures in Asian studies. Protrusion of an aortic cusp into the VSD is exceptional: It occurred in only 3 of 19 patients with associated AI. The anatomic substrate of the aortic leak is variable and cusps not adjacent to the VSD are often involved. Severely deformed aortic valves were found in the two oldest patients. The results of VSD closure and aortic valvuloplasty are encouraging when the operation is performed in childhood.

Ventricular septal defect in Chinese with aortic valve prolapse and aortic regurgitation*

Hung-Chi Lue, Tseng-Chen Sung, Shou-Hsien Hou, Mei-Hwan Wu, Su-Ju Cheng, Shu-Hsung Chu, and Chi-Ren Hung

Aortic regurgitation (AR) is one of the most important complications occurring in patients with ventricular septal defect (VSD). It occurred in 1.9%–5.5% of all patients with VSD in Western countries [1-6] but occurred at higher rates, 7.0%–13.1%, in Hawaii [7] and Japan [8, 9], suggesting that a racial difference exists. Aortic valve prolapse might, as proposed by Blumenthal et al. [10] in 1967, precede the development of AR, particularly in patients with subpulmonic VSD. Whether Chinese, like Japanese, are prone to develop aortic valve prolapse and AR is unknown [11]. Controversies still exist regarding the optimal surgical treatment and timing of the operation for such patients due to a paucity of information [1, 5, 12-16]. To clarify these matters, we started in January, 1978 a prospective study to identify the anatomical type of the VSD and to check the integrity and competency of the aortic valves of all infants and children with VSD to be catheterized at the National Taiwan University Hospital. Another 306 patients with VSD who were catheterized from 1970 to 1977 were also reviewed to determine the type of VSD and the integrity and competency of the aortic valve. An analysis of the results of these two studies forms the basis of this report.

Materials and methods

Prospective study

From January 1978 to June 1983, 375 infants and children with VSD as an isolated or prime lesion consecutively catheterized at the National Taiwan University Hospital were subjected to this prospective study. With the informed consent of parents, simultaneous pressures in the systemic and pulmonary arteries as well as oxygen saturations in each chamber of the heart were measured, and angiocardiograms were obtained. The contrast medium was injected through a ventriculography or NIH catheter (no. 6 to no. 9) placed in the left ventricle and also in the portion immediately above the aortic valve. The cinefilm speed was set at 60 frames/s. Thus, in each of 361 consecutive patients, left ventricular and aortic root cineangiocardiograms of the frontal and lateral projections (Philips Poly Diagnost C and Optimus M 200 generator) were obtained. Axial cineangiograms of the four-chamber view and long axial oblique view were obtained as needed,

* This paper appeared in Heart and Vessels Vol. 2, No. 2 (1986).
Address reprint request to: Hung-Chi Lue, M.D., No. 1, Chang-teh St., National Taiwan University Hospital, Taipei, Taiwan, R.O.C. 100

starting in 1982 [17-19]. The patients' ages ranged from 1 month to 19 years, mean 7.5 years (Table 1). Patients with VSD with severe infundibular stenosis, atrioventricular and/or ventriculoarterial discordance, and perforation of the coronary cusp due to bacterial endocarditis were excluded. The general type of the VSD was determined and the appearance and mobility of the coronary cusps and sinus of Valsalva and valve competency were assessed.

Retrospective study

Another 306 infants and children who had VSD as an isolated lesion were reviewed. AOT Elema-Schoenander biplane left ventriculography (306 cases) and aortography (88 cases) were carried out in these patients from January 1970 to December 1977. Their ages ranged from 5 months to 16 years, mean 5.6 years (Table 1). The type of VSD and the integrity and competency of the aortic valve were similarly checked.

Diagnostic criteria for the general type of VSD

The VSD was identified and classified, mainly on the basis of left ventriculograms of lateral projection, into four general types [16-20]: (1) Subpulmonic VSD: Visualization of a shunt from the left ventricle to the right ventricular outflow tract above the membranous septum and the crista supraventricularis, which appeared as a lucent zone between the right coronary sinus of Valsalva and the posterior border of the infundibulum (Fig. 1) [17]. Included in this general type of subpulmonic VSD were the subarterial outlet and muscular outlet types of VSD [16-20]. (2) Subaortic VSD: An opacified shunt from the left ventricle to the body or outflow tract of the right ventricle through the membranous septum just below the right sinus of Valsalva and the crista supraventricularis (Fig. 2) [16, 17]. (3) Atrioventricular canal VSD: An opacified shunt through the defect involving both membranous and muscular inlet septa in proximity to the atrioventricular valves [16-19]. Usually, ECG showed abnormal atrioventricular conduction [16, 19]. (4) Muscular VSD: A shunt across the muscular inlet or trabecular septum below the membranous septum with separation from the mitral annulus [16].

Diagnostic criteria for aortic valve prolapse and AR

Based mainly on the lateral view of aortic root angiograms, prolapse of the right and noncoronary cusp and sinus was identified [8, 21]. A protrusion appeared beyond the natural contour of the right, noncoronary cusp and the sinus of Valsalva, forming a double shadow, more marked at the early and midsystolic phases if the cusp and sinus

Table 1. Overall incidence of aortic valve prolapse and AR in VSD

Patient series (years of study)	No. of cases	Age in years (mean)	AR	Prolapse without AR	Total
Prospective (1978-1983)	361	1/12-19 (7.5)	20 (5.5)[a]	23 (6.4)	43 (11.9)
Retrospective (1970-1977)	306	5/12-16 (5.6)	22 (7.2)[b]	15 (4.9)	37 (12.1)
Total	667	1/12-19	42 (6.3)	38 (5.7)	80 (12.0)

[a] Including three patients with bicuspid aortic valve
[b] Including one patient with bicuspid aortic valve

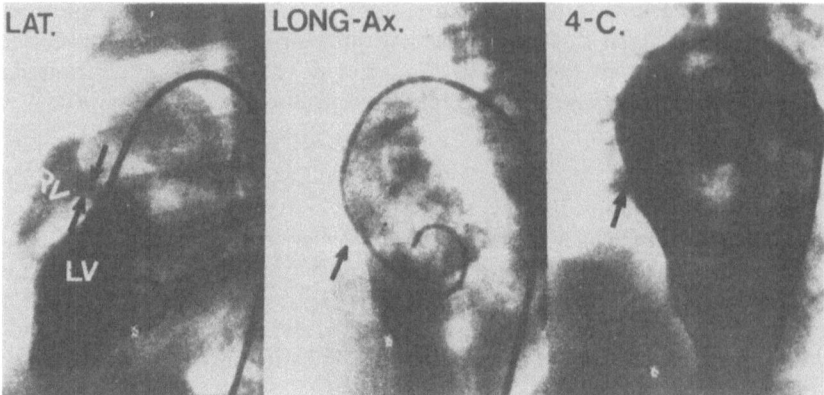

Fig. 1. Selective left ventriculograms of lateral (*LAT.*) long-axis oblique (*LONG-Ax.*) and four-chamber (*4-C.*) views. A subpulmonic VSD is best seen with the lateral view, below the pulmonary valve, and above a lucent zone of the crista supraventricularis

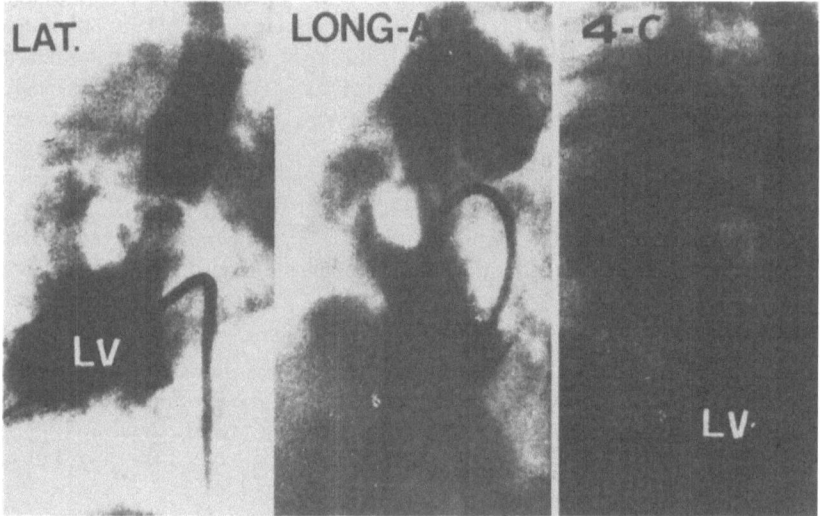

Fig. 2. Selective left ventriculograms of lateral (*LAT.*), long-axis oblique (*LONG-Ax.*), and four-chamber (*4-C.*) views, showing a subaortic VSD below the aortic valve and a lucent zone of crista suproventricularis (*asterisk*)

were still mobile (Fig. 3) [8, 9, 21]. The degree of AR was determined as mild, moderate, or severe based on aortic root angiography [22].

Follow-up studies

Open-heart closure of the VSD alone, or with valvuloplasty or replacement of the aortic valve, was carried out; the pathological condition was checked at each surgical interven-

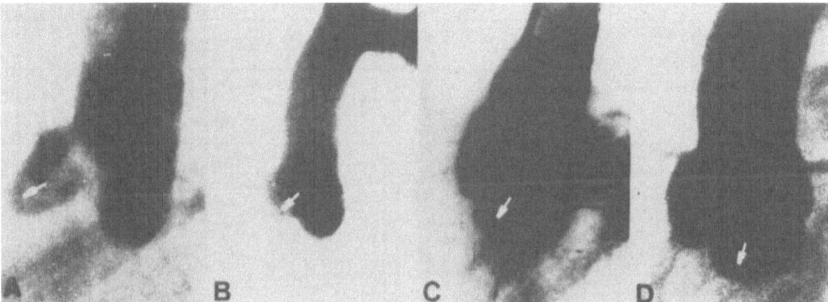

Fig. 3 A-D. Selective aortic root angiograms of lateral projection showing a spectrum of prolapsed coronary sinus of Valsalva and cusps. **A** Right coronary sinus of Valsalva and cusp prolapsed without AR in subpulmonic VSD. **B** Right coronary cusp prolapsed without AR in subaortic VSD. **C** Right and noncoronary cusps prolapsed with mild AR in subaortic VSD. **D** Noncoronary cusp prolapsed with mild AR in subaortic VSD

tion. All patients were followed-up at the cardiac clinic; follow-up cardiac catheterization was advised and carried out.

Statistical analysis

The incidence of aortic valve prolapse and/or AR among the series of patients was compared for statistical significance using the χ^2 test or Yates' continuity correction.

Results

Overall incidence of aortic valve prolapse and AR

Prospective study. Of the 361 consecutive VSD patients studied, 43 (11.9%) had valve prolapse and/or AR: 20 patients (5.5%) were with AR and 23 (6.4%) had valve prolapse without AR (Table 1). The aortic valve was bicuspid in three patients.

Retrospective study. Of the 306 patients reviewed, 37 (12.1%) had the valve complication: 22 patients (7.2%) were with AR, and 15 (4.9%) had prolapse without AR (Table 1). Of those patients with AR, one had a bicuspid aortic valve.

A total of 80 patients with the valve complication were thus identified from the 667 patients of the two study groups. The overall incidence of aortic valve prolapse and AR was 12.0%. Sixty patients were males and 20 females, indicating a male preponderance.

VSD types and aortic valve prolapse and AR

In 332 of 361 consecutive patients prospectively studied, the type of VSD was determined: 75 (22.6%) were subpulmonic VSD, 249 (75.0%) were the subaortic type, including atrioventricular septal defect, and there were 37 others, including three (0.9%) cases of artrioventricular canal VSD, two (0.6%) muscular inlet or trabecular VSD, and three (0.9%) multiple VSD (Table 2). Aortic valve prolapse and AR occurred in 21 (28.0%) cases of subpulmonic VSD and in 22 (8.8%) cases of subaortic VSD ($P < 0.005$). No valve lesions were observed in the 37 other patients.

Table 2. VSD type and incidence of aortic valve prolapse and AR, prospective study (1978–1983)

Aortic valve	Type of VSD			
	Subpulmonic ($n = 75$)	Subaortic ($n = 249$)	Other ($n = 37$)	All types ($n = 361$)
Normal	52 (69.3)	224 (90.0)	30 (81.1)	306 (84.8)
Prolapse and AR	21 (28.0)[a]	22 (8.8)[a]		43 (11.9)
AR	8 (1[b])	12 (2[b])		20 (5.5)
	(10.7)	(4.8)		
Prolapse	13 (17.3)	10 (4.0)		23 (6.4)
Undetermined	2 (2.7)	3 (1.2)	7 (18.9)	12 (3.3)

Others including atrioventricular canal VSD (three cases), trabeculated VSD (two), multiple VSD (three), and type undetermined (29)
[a] Test for difference ($P < 0.005$)
[b] Bicuspid aortic valve

Age of development of valve complications

The age distribution of the 80 VSD patients with valve prolapse and AR is shown in Fig. 4. Of the 49 patients with subpulmonic VSD, the youngest age of prolapse was 7 months and of AR was 3 years 8 months. Of the 31 cases of subaortic VSD, the youngest ages of prolapse and AR were 2 years and 3 years 6 months, respectively. The patients with AR were older in general than those with prolapse. Valve prolapse occurred mostly before the age of 6–10 years, leading progressively to AR.

Changes in coronary cusps and sinus of Valsalva·

The coronary cusps prolapsed in 49 patients with subpulmonic VSD were limited to the right cusp. No such prolapsed cusp appeared on aortic root angiocardiograms in two cases (Table 3). The cusps involved in 31 patients with subaortic VSD were either the right, noncoronary, or both right and noncoronary cusps, which appeared as prolapsed

Table 3. Coronary cusps prolapsed in subpulmonic and subaortic VSD

Type of VSD and cusps prolapsed	No. of cases	Percentage
Subpulmonic VSD	49	61.3
RCC, without AR	32 (1[a])	40.0
with AR	15	18.8
Nonprotruding, with AR	2 (1[b])	2.5
Subaortic VSD	31	38.7
RCC, without AR	11	13.7
with AR	2 (1[a])	2.5
NCC, without AR	2	2.5
with AR	1 (1[a])	1.3
RCC and NCC, without AR	2	2.5
with AR	7	8.7
Nonprotruding, with AR	6 (1[a], 3[+])	7.5
Total	80	100.0

RCC right coronary cusp, *NCC* noncoronary cusp
[a] Associated with infundibular stenosis
[b] Bicuspid aortic valve

on aortograms in all but six cases. Of the six patients with AR showing no prolapse on angiocardiograms, four were with bicuspid aortic valve. The cusps were mobile and competent in 46 patients (Table 4). Various degrees of valve prolapse and AR occurred in the remaining patients. In a 14-year-old girl with subaortic VSD, the aneurysmally dilated right sinus of Valsalva ruptured into the right ventricle, where sagging of the right coronary cusp was mild, leading to no regurgitation.

Hemodynamics and size of VSD

In 69 patients with cusp prolapse and AR, simultaneous systemic and pulmonary artery pressures were measured (Table 5). The mean pulmonary artery pressure was below 20

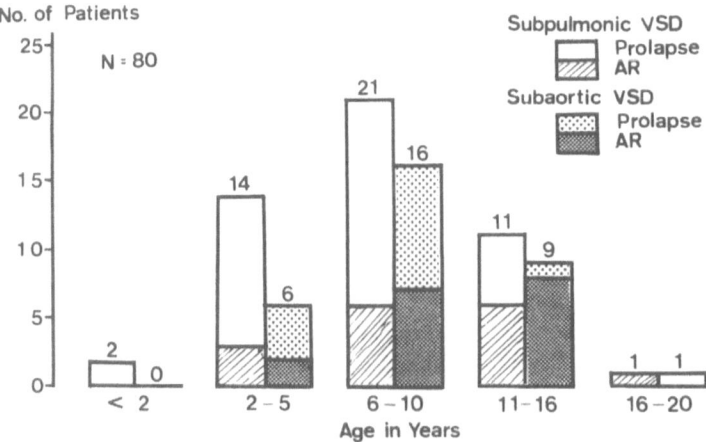

Fig. 4. The number of VSD patients with aortic valve prolapse and aortic regurgitation (*AR*). Valve complications occurred earlier in those with subpulmonic than with subaortic VSD, most frequently in patients aged 6–10 years

Table 4. Severity of aortic valve prolapse and AR

Severity of aortic valve prolapse	Subpulmonic VSD	Subaortic VSD	All
Mobile, without AR	32 (65.3)[a]	14 (45.2)	46 (57.5)
Mobile, mild AR	5 (10.2)	5 (16.1)[a]	10 (12.5)
Poorly mobile, with moderate AR	8 (16.3)	5 (16.1)[a]	13 (16.3)
Not mobile, severe AR or rupture	2 (4.1)	1 (3.2)[b]	3 (3.7)
Nonprotruding, mild to severe AR	2 (4.1)[c]	6 (19.4)[a, d]	8 (10.0)
All groups (%)	49 (100.0)	31 (100.0)	80 (100.0)

[a] One case each with mild to moderate infundibular stenosis
[b] Ruptured sinus of Valsalva
[c] One patient with bicuspid aortic valve
[d] Three patients with bicuspid aortic valve

Table 5. Hemodynamic data for VSD with aortic valve prolapse and AR

Severity of aortic valve prolapse	Mean PA pressure < 20 mmHg		Mean PA pressure ≥ 20 mmHg		Total No. of cases
	Qp/Qs <1.5	Qp/Qs >1.5	Rp/Rs <0.2	Rp/Rs 0.2-0.49	
Mobile, without AR	22	10	1	6	39
Mobile, mild AR	7	1	1	1	10
Poorly mobile, with moderate AR	5	4	3	—	12
Not mobile, severe AR or rupture	—	—	—	2	2
Nonprotruding, mild to severe AR	5	—	1	—	6
Total	39	15	6	9	69
(%)	(56.5)	(21.7)	(8.7)	(13.1)	(100.0)

PA pulmonary artery, *Qp/Qs* pulmonary to systemic flow ratio, *Rp/Rs* pulmonary to systemic resistance ratio

mmHg in more than two-thirds of the patients. The magnitude of left-to-right shunts was small in 39 (56.5%) patients. The pulmonary resistance was almost always normal but mildly elevated in only nine (13.1%) patients. The average diameter of the subpulmonic VSD measured at surgery in 37 patients ranged from 0.5 to 1.5 cm, with a mean of 0.99 ± 0.37 cm. The diameter of the subaortic VSD in 29 patients ranged from 0.4 to 2.0 cm, mean 1.05 ± 0.42 cm. In the subpulmonic type of VSD, the prolapsed cusp almost always partially or completely occluded the defect.

Follow-up and outcome

Of the 80 patients with valve lesions, 72 underwent open-heart closure of the VSD. Valvuloplasty was carried out in ten patients with subpulmonic VSD and in five of the subaortic type. Valve replacement was performed in two patients with subpulmonic VSD and in another patient with subaortic VSD, whose valves were either severely deformed or bicuspid. All survived, and ten patients were recatheterized.

Discussion

Specific identification of a VSD as one of the four general types — subpulmonic, subaortic, atrioventricular canal, and muscular VSD — has become possible, based on angiocardiographic data. Selective left ventriculography of the lateral, long-axial oblique, and four-chamber views has proved to be a main and reliable diagnostic procedure. Aortic root cineangiocardiography, especially of the lateral projection, is most useful in the evaluation of the integrity and competency of the aortic valve in VSD [8, 9, 21]. The aortograms may fail to show a cusp prolapse due to a bicuspid aortic valve or other reasons, as happened in 8 (10%) of 80 patients we studied. The lateral profile of the right sinus of Valsalva and its cusp usually appeared round and with a smooth contour on angiograms, but it frequently also appeared angular, triangular, square with or without a notch, or round with an indentation. In some cases, this mimicked coronary cusp prolapse, requiring surgical confirmation (unpublished observation). Careful examination of the contour and its cusp motion during the cardiac cycle on cineangiograms usually suffices for the diagnosis.

Our prospective study indicated that Chinese, like Japanese, have a higher incidence of subpulmonic VSD and are more prone to develop aortic valve complications than are Occidentals (Table 6) [1-9]. In a prospective study, Tatsuno et al. [9] found a very high incidence (41.7%) of valve prolapse in 24 patients with asymptomatic subpulmonic VSD, aged 4-27 years. A high incidence of 35.7%, comparable with that among Japanese ($P < 0.1$), was also noted in the present study among 137 patients with subpulmonic VSD (Table 6). The development of the conal septum in Orientals may, as Ando [28] suspected, differ from that in Occidentals. The frequent occurrence of valve lesions in subpulmonic VSD could result from the inherent structural abnormality, leaving the right sinus of Valsalva and coronary cusp unsupported by the conal septum from below [15]; in part it may be caused by hemodynamic impacts, so-called Venturi effects, and the Bernoulli principle, generated by the left-to-right shunting through the defect [21]. The prolapsed aortic cusp herniating into the right ventricular outflow tract may appear as a balloon and cause a significant obstruction [24]. Van Praagh and McNamara [15] found in 1968 that in patients with subaortic VSD the aortic valve became prolapsed and even with AR due to altered hemodynamics and faulty valve commissures or leaflet opposition.

The age of onset of the diastolic murmur indicating AR as reported in the literature ranged from 6 months to 9 years [14], 6 months to 14 years [7], and 2 to 8 years [27]. The youngest patient with valve complications ever reported was 6 months old; the oldest was 57 years. The majority of patients were between 6 and 16 years [7, 12, 14, 27]. The aortic valve may, as shown in the present study, start to prolapse during infancy and early childhood, reaching a peak by the age of 6-10 years. Blumenthal et al. [10] and Tatsuno et al. [9] suggested that the prolapsed cusp and sinus of Valsalva might deteriorate and proceed to AR. The incidence of valve complications in VSD varied therefore with age. The time interval needed for the prolapsed cusp to progress to AR remains controversial. Rupture of the sinus of Valsalva occurs usually in late childhood and or in adulthood [26]. Whether or not rupture of the sinus of Valsalva is the terminal event of cusp prolapse related to VSD still remains conjectural. In our series of patients, there was only one such patient in whom no AR was demonstrated. It is likely that wall factors, such as

Table 6. Incidence of aortic valve prolapse and AR in VSD in variouus countries

Countries, authors, year	No. of VSD patients studied	Ages [years]	AR		Prolapse without AR		Total	
			No.	Percent	No.	Percent	No.	Percent
USA, Nadas et al., 1964 [1]	756	3-29	34	4.5	—	—	—	—
1972 [2]	2059	3-29	60	2.9[b]	—	—	—	—
Cooley et al., 1962 [3]	300[a]	0-49	8	2.7[b]	—	—	—	—
Karapawich et al., 1981 [4]	1692	All	32	1.9[b]	—	—	—	—
Keane et al., 1977 [5]	1265	2-41	69	5.5	—	—	—	—
Denmark, Andersen and Lomholt, 1972 [6]	203	All	6	3.1	—	—	—	—
Hawaii, Moreno-Cabral et al., 1976 [7]	357	All	25	7.0	—	—	—	—
Japan, Tatsuno et al., 1973 [8]	1108[a]	All	91	8.2	—	—	—	—
1975 [9]	551[a]	All	72	13.1[b]	—	—	—	—
subpulmonic VSD, 1975 [9]	24	4-27	—	—	10	41.7	10	41.7[c]
Taiwan, 1970-1983, present study	667	1/12-19	42	6.3	38	5.7	80	12.0
subpulmonic VSD 1970-1983	137	1/12-19	17	12.4	32	23.4	49	35.7

[a] Surgical series
[b] $P < 0.01$ compared with prospective and retrospective series combined in Taiwan
[c] $P > 0.1$ compared with subpulmonic VSD series in Taiwan

dysplasia or interruption of the tunica media muscle fibers, may have been present [25]. Most of the mortality occurred in untreated patients at about age 20 [23]. All patients with subpulmonic VSD with cusp prolapse and AR were advised by us to undergo surgery soon after the diagnosis was made, or at least before the age of 5 years, as recommended by Karapawich et al. [4]. Following surgery, in five of our patients with subpulmonic VSD and AR, the diastolic murmur disappeared and the prolapsed cusp returned to its normal position, as observed by Chung and Manning [27]. This kind of normalizing process was not apparent in patients with subaortic VSD. A new regurgitation murmur developed in two patients following surgical closure of the subaortic VSD and in another patient whose subaortic VSD had spontaneously closed.

Conclusion

The incidence of aortic valve prolapse and aortic regurgitation (AR) among Chinese with ventricular septal defect (VSD) has not been studied, and controversies still exist regarding optimal surgical treatment and timing of operation for this condition. A prospective study of 332 consecutive patients with VSD showed that aortic valve prolapse and AR occurred in 43 (11.9%) patients. Valve lesions occurred more commonly among patients with subpulmonic VSD (28.0%) than with subaortic VSD (8.8%) ($P < 0.005$). A retrospective study of another 306 patients revealed that 37 (12.1%) had valve complications. Of the 80 patients with valve lesions, 60 were males and 20 were females. The youngest ages of prolapse and AR in subpulmonic VSD were 7 months and 3 years 8 months, respectively; those in subaortic VSD were 2 years and 3 years 6 months, respectively. Valve prolapse occurred mostly before the age of 6–10 years, leading progressively to AR. The coronary cusps prolapsed in subpulmonic VSD were limited to the right cusp; and those in subaortic VSD were the right cusp, noncoronary cusp, or both. The magnitude of left-to-right shunts was small and the pulmonary artery pressure was normal in the majority of patients. Seventy-two patients underwent open-heart closure of the VSD, with additional valvuloplasty in 15 and valve replacement in three patients. It is concluded that Chinese with VSD are prone to develop aortic valve complications. Surgical closure of the subpulmonic VSD may restore the prolapsed valve to normal. Closure of the subaortic VSD has little effect. Valvuloplasty in subaortic VSD may palliate AR, but in all probability cannot restore valve competency.

References

1. Nadas AS, Thilenius OG, LaFarge CG, Hauck AJ (1964) Ventricular septal defect with aortic regurgitation: Medical and pathologic aspects. Circulation 29: 862–873
2. Nadas AS, Fyler DC (1972) Ventricular septal defect with aortic regurgitation. In: Nadas AS (ed) Pediatric cardiology (3rd edn). Saunders, Philadelphia, p 379
3. Cooley DA, Garrett HE, Howard HS (1962) The surgical treatment of ventricular septal defect: An analysis of 300 consecutive surgical cases. Prog Cardiovasc Dis 4: 312–323
4. Karapawich PP, Duff DF, Mullins CE, Cooley DA et al (1981) Ventricular septal defect with associated aortic valve insufficiency: Progression of insufficiency and operative results in young children. J Thorac Cardiovasc Surg 82: 182–189
5. Keane JF, Plauth WH, Nadas AS (1977) Ventricular septal defect with aortic regurgitation. Circulation (Suppl) 56: 72–77
6. Andersen HK, Lomholt P (1972) Ventricular septal defect and aortic insufficiency. Scand J Thorac Cardiovasc Surg 6: 57–67
7. Moreno-Cabral RJ, Mamiya RT, Nakamura FF (1977) Ventricular septal defect and aortic insufficiency. J Thorac Cardiovasc Surg 73: 358–365

8. Tatsuno K, Konno S, Sakakibara S (1973) Ventricular septal defect with aortic insufficiency: Angio-cardiographic aspects and a new classification. Am Heart J 85: 13-21
9. Tatsuno K, Ando M, Takao A, Hatsune K, Konno S (1975) Diagnostic importance of aortography in conal ventricular septal defect. Am Heart J 89: 171-177
10. Blumenthal S, Malm JR, Ellis K (1967) Natural history of ventricular septal defect with aortic valve prolapse (Abstract). Circulation 35, 36: II-73
11. Lue HC (1986) This volume, pp 3-8
12. Winchell P, Bashour F (1956) Ventricular septal defect with aortic incompetence simulating patent ductus arteriosus. Am J Med 361-365
13. Plauth WH, Braunwald E, Rockoff SD (1965) Ventricular septal defect and aortic regurgitation: Clinical, hemodynamic and surgical considerations. Am J Med 39: 552-567
14. Halloran KH, Talner NS, Browne MJ (1965) A study of ventricular septal defect associated with aortic insufficiency. 69: 320-327
15. Starr A, Menashe V, Dotter C (1960) Surgical correction of aortic insufficiency associated with ventricular septal defect. Surg Gynecol Obstet 71-77
16. Van Praagh R, McNamara JJ (1968) Anatomic types of ventricular septal defect with aortic insufficiency: Diagnostic and surgical considerations. Am Heart J 75: 604-619
17. Baron MG, Wolf BS, Steinfeld L (1968) Angiographic diagnosis of subpulmonic ventricular septal defect. Am J Roentgenol 103: 93-103
18. Bargeron LM Jr, Elliot LP, Soto B, Bream PR, Curry GC (1977) Axial cineangiography in congenital heart disease. Section I, Concept, technical and anatomical considerations. Circulation 56: 1075-83
19. Green CE, Elliot LP, Bargeron LM Jr (1981) Axial cineangiographic evaluation of the posterior ventricular septal defect. Am J Cardiol 48: 331-335
20. Steinfeld L, Dimich I, Park SC, Baron MG (1972) Clinical diagnosis of isolated subpulmonic (supra-cristal) ventricular septal defect. Am J Cardiol 30: 19-24
21. Tatsuno K, Konno S, Ando M, Sakakibara S (1973) Pathogetic mechanisms of prolapsing aortic valve and aortic regurgitation associated with ventricular septal defect. Anatomical, angiographic, and surgical considerations. Circulation 48: 1028-37
22. Lehman J, Boyle J, Debbas J (1962) Quantitation of aortic valvular insufficiency by catheter thoracic angiography. Radiology 79: 361-369
23. Keith JD, Rowe RD, Vlad P (1978) Heart disease in infancy and childhood. (3rd edn). Macmillan, New York, pp 320-321
24. Jaffe RB, Scherer JL (1977) Supracristal ventricular septal defects: Spectrum of associated lesions and complications. Am J Roentgenol 128: 629-637
25. Edwards JE, Burchell HB (1957) The pathological anatomy of deficiencies between the aortic root and the heart, including aortic sinus aneurysms. Thorax 12: 125-139
26. Sakakibara S, Konno S (1962) Congenital aneurysms of sinus of Valsalva. A clinical study. Am Heart J 63: 708-719
27. Chung KJ, Manning JA (1974) Ventricular septal defect associated with aortic insufficiency: Medical and surgical management. Am Heart J 87: 435-438
28. Ando M (1974) Letters to the editor: Subpulmonary ventricular septal defect with pulmonary stenosis. Circulation 50: 412-413

Treatment of ventricular septal defect and coronary cusp prolapse

Surgery of ventricular septal defect with prolapse of aortic cusp

Chi-Ren Hung

Controversy still exists as to the surgical indication of subpulmonic or type 1 ventricular septal defect (VSD-I), particularly when it causes only small left-to-right shunts. Efforts have been focused on whether or not VSD-I has a high incidence of combined prolapsed aortic cusp, which may lead to aortic regurgitation, or if closure of the VSD-I is effective in preventing the prolapse of the aortic cusp and aortic regurgitation. There are also differences of opinion with regard to when to operate and these should be resolved. The purpose of this communication is to report on patients with VSD who underwent operation at the Department of Surgery of National Taiwan University Hospital and to try and reach answers to the above problems.

Materials

Between January 1964 and June 1983, a total of 564 patients with VSD were operated upon at National Taiwan University Hospital. All patients were catheterized and the diagnosis was based on both clinical and angiocardiographic findings. Of these, 323 cases were males (57.3%) and 241 (42.7%) females. The male to female ratio was 1.3:1. There were 194 cases of subpulmonic or type I VSD (34.4%), 355 cases (62.9%) of type II or membranous type VSD (VSD-II), 11 cases (2.0%) of type III (VSD-III) and four cases (0.7%) of type IV (VSD-IV) or VSD at the muscular portion of the septum (Table 1). The age ranged from 3 months to 63 years. There is an increase in the number of cases of VSD-I with age: 28% in patients below 1 year of age; 50% in patients older than 30 years of age.

Table 1. Age, sex, and type of VSD (1964–1983, National Taiwan University Hospital, $n = 564$)

Age [years]	Sex		Type of VSD			
	Male	Female	I	II	III	IV
0–1	16(57.1%)	12(42.1%)	8(28.6%)	20(71.4%)	0	0
2–5	56(58.3%)	40(41.7%)	21(21.9%)	72(75.0%)	3(3.1%)	0
6–10	95(55.9%)	75(44.1%)	51(30.0%)	116(68.2%)	0	3(1.8%)
11–20	78(51.3%)	74(48.7%)	63(41.4%)	83(54.6%)	6(4.0%)	0
21–30	58(65.9%)	30(34.1%)	36(40.9%)	49(55.7%)	2(2.3%)	1(1.1%)
Total	323(57.3%)	241(42.7%)	194(34.4%)	355(62.9%)	11(2.0%)	4(0.7%)

Operation

All patients were operated under cardiopulmonary bypass with moderate hypothermia and in six cases of infants below the age of 1 year, the technique of deep hypothermia and total circulatory arrest was used for repair of the VSD. After 1978, a cardioplegic solution was utilized for intraoperative myocardial protection.

For VSD-I, repair of the VSD was originally made through right ventriculotomy; for the past 2 years, however, the approach to the VSD has been made through the main pulmonary artery. VSD-II was repaired either through right ventriculotomy or right atriotomy. Prolapse of the aortic cusp without aortic regurgitation was not dealt with during surgery and when it was associated with aortic regurgitation, a reconstructive procedure was carried out through aortotomy. The technique of the reconstructive procedure on the aortic cusp was to approximate the edge of the three aortic cusps at the region of the central nodules of each cusp by a 5-0 prolene stay suture. The redundunt cusps were plicated and anchored at the level of the commissures to the outside of the aortic wall by mattress sutures.

Operative mortality

There were nine mortalities among 194 cases of VSD-I (4.6% operative mortality), 28 mortalities among 355 cases of VSD-II (7.9% operative mortality), two mortalities among 11 cases of VSD-III (18% operative mortality), and one mortality among four cases of VSD-IV (25% operative mortality).

Relations between the type of VSD and aortic valvular lesions. An analysis was made to determine whether the type of VSD affects or induces aortic cusp lesions such as prolapse, regurgitation, and/or ruptured aneurysm of the sinus of Valsalva (RASV). Of the 194 cases of VSD-I, 114 cases or 58.8% were associated with aortic cusp lesions, i.e., 18 cases or 9.3% were associated with RASV, 49 cases or 25% were found on aortograms to have prolapse of the right coronary cusp, and 47 cases or 24.2% were found to be associated with aortic regurgitation (AR). In 355 cases of VSD-II, only 20 cases or 5.6% were associated with aortic cusp lesions, i.e. three cases or 0.8% with RASV, six cases of 1.7% with prolapse of the aortic cusp (noncoronary cusp), and 11 cases or 3.1% with AR.

The incidence of combination of aortic valvular lesions was much higher in VSD-I than in VSD-II. Furthermore, the incidence of combined aortic valvular lesions in VSD-I increased with age: Only one case or 12.5% of patients below 1 year of age was found to have combined aortic cusp prolapse, whereas this incidence increased to 38.1% in the age-group of 2-5 years, 49.0% in the age-group 6-10 years, 65.0% in the age-group 11-20 years, 75.0% in the age-group 21-30 years, and as high as 80.0% in patients older than 31 years.

In this series, the youngest VSD-I patient combined with AR was 4 years and the youngest VSD-I patient with RASV was 16 years old. The incidence of combined aortic cusp lesion was not remarkable among VSD-II patients (Table 2).

It is noteworthy that the incidence of combined RASV became more prominent in the older age-group; 7.9% among the age-group 11-20 years but 33.3% of patients with VSD-I above the age of 31 years had combined RASV (Table 2).

The patients were divided into four subgroups. Group 1 consisted of cases with closure of the VSD with angiographic evidence of prolapse of the aortic cusp only, without aortic regurgitation (Table 3). Group 2 were the cases of VSD with mild aortic regurgitation for

Table 2. Type of VSD and aortic lesion (1964–1983, National Taiwan University Hospital, $n = 564$)

Age [years]	VSD I					VSD II				
	No.	RASV[a]	AR[b]	Prolapse	Total	No.	RASV	AR	Prolapse	Total
0-1	8	0	0	1 (12.5%)	1 (12.5%)	20	0	0	0	0
2-5	21	0	3 (14.3%)	5 (23.8%)	8 (38.1%)	72	0	0	1 (1.4%)	1 (1.4%)
6-10	51	0	7 (13.7%)	18 (35.3%)	25 (49.0%)	116	0	4 (3.4%)	2 (1.7%)	6 (5.2%)
11-20	63	5 (7.9%)	22 (34.9%)	14 (22.2%)	41 (65.0%)	83	0	4 (4.8%)	3 (3.6%)	7 (8.4%)
21-30	36	8 (22.2%)	12 (33.3%)	7 (19.5%)	27 (75.0%)	49	2 (4.1%)	2 (4.1%)	0	4 (8.2%)
31-63	15	5 (33.3%)	3 (20.0%)	4 (26.7%)	12 (80.0%)	15	1 (6.7%)	1 (6.7%)	0	2 (13.4%)
Total	194	18 (9.3%)	47 (24.2%)	49 (25.3%)	114 (58.8%)	355	3 (0.8%)	11 (3.1%)	6 (1.7%)	20 (5.6%)

[a] Including RASV and prolapse
[b] Including AR and RASV

Table 3. Early and late VSD closure only for VSD with prolapse (group 1)

	No. of cases	Early	Late	Follow-up duration	
				Mean	Range
VSD-I	48	0/48	2/48	64 mo	9 mo – 9 yr 3 mo
VSD-II	5	0/5	1/5	40 mo	1 yr 7 mo – 5 yr
VSD-III	1	0/1	0/1	20 mo	

which patch repair of the VSD was performed and aortic regurgitation was left alone (Table 4). Group 3 included cases of VSD with aortic regurgitation of moderate of severe degree; aortic valvuloplasty was done in addition to patch repair of VSD (Table 5). Group 4 were the cases in which valvuloplasty for aortic valve was unsuccessful and aortic valve replacement had to be carried out in addition to patch closure of VSD (Table 6).

Group 1 consisted of 48 cases of VSD-1, five cases of VSD-II, and one case of VSD-III followed-up for 9 months to 9 years 3 months, mean 64 months (Table 3). There were no AR murmurs in the early postoperative period (during hospitalization). Two cases, a 25-year-old male and a 29-year-old male, developed AR murmur during the late follow-up period. Among five cases of VSD-II, one case developed a late AR murmur. Obviously, in the two VSD-I cases, repair of VSD-I had not prevented the prolapsed cusps to progress to AR. But if compared with the total incidence of VSD-I plus AR in this series of 24.2% (Table 2), it may be said that the incidence of progress to AR in repaired VSD-I was less.

Deformed aortic cusp in the older patients may have been responsible for the progress to AR.

Group 2 consisted of 13 patients with VSD-I and one with VSD-II (Table 4). In this group, only VSD repair was done and the aortic valve was left alone. AR murmur, which was present before surgery, disappeared in five cases postoperatively. Repair of VSD-I only helped to reduce mild AR and made the aortic valve become competent.

Table 4. Early and late AR after VSD closure only for VSD and mild AR (group 2)

	No. of cases	Early	Late	Follow-up duration	
				Mean	Range
VSD-I	13	4/13	4/11[a]	75 mo	8 mo – 9 yr 10 mo
VSD-II	1	1/1	1/1	16 mo	

[a] Two early mortalities

Table 5. Early and late AR after VSD closure and valvoplasty for VSD and AR (group 3)

	No. of cases	Early	Late	Follow-up duration	
				Mean	Range
VSD-I	17	8/17	8/17	39 mo	6 mo – 7 yr 2 mo
VSD-II	5	4/5	4/5	38 mo	9 mo – 7 yr 4 mo
VSD-III	2	1/2	1/2	45 mo	3 yr 4 mo – 4 yr 2 mo

Group 3 consisted of 17 cases of VSD-I, five cases of VSD-II, and two cases of VSD-III (Table 5). In addition to patch repair of the VSD, aortic valvuloplasty was always attempted to produce a competent valve as judged by the absence of diastolic regurgitation thrill after the patient came off the cardiopulmonary bypass. AR murmur recurred in 7 of 19 cases of VSD-I in the early postoperative period and was persistent in 7 of 13 cases during the late follow-up period. The AR recurrence rate was high in VSD-II patients — seven of eight cases showed recurrence.

We observed in this group of patients that the aortic valve leaflet which became incompetent was no longer normal in appearance.

The aortic cusp which was most involved, such as the right coronary cusp in VSD-I patients, was thickened, fibrotic, and redundant. Whether this abnormal cusp will be able to come into good coaptation and become competent with the other two cusps in the long run after valvuloplasty is uncertain. It is also possible that this fibrotic change, once obtained, could be progressive and be responsible for the recurrence of AR after reconstructive repair. From the observations we made from these groups, the question arises: Should we postpone the repair of VSD-I until AR appears simply because hemodynamic studies show the VSD-I to have a small left-to-right shunt? In other words, should we delay the small VSD-I closure until the aortic valve has become abnormal enough to produce AR? We have to accept the fact that repair of an abnormal aortic valve to maintain its long-term competency is not very successful. Furthermore, it is frequently seen during surgery that a hemodynamically small VSD-I may be an anatomically large VSD-I because the VSD is partially or almost totally occluded by the prolapsed aortic cusp. We also noted that the prolapsed cusp, although still competent, was already thickened in a 10-month-old baby.

Group 4 consisted of 17 cases of VSD-I and five cases of VSD-II (Table 6). All patients received aortic valve replacement because of the failure to reconstruct the competent valve. There has been no recurrence of AR murmur except for one patient in whom AR murmur was found 43 months after surgery but who died suddenly before further management could be undertaken.

Table 6. Early and late AR after VSD repair and AVR for VSD and AR (group 4)

	No. of cases	Early	Late	Follow-up duration	
				Mean	Range
VSD-I	17	0/17	1/15[a]	48 mo	8 mo – 7 yr 6 mo
VSD-II	5	0/5	0/5	51 mo	1 yr 4 mo – 8 yr 4 mo

[a] Two early mortalities. One AR case was detected and died suddenly 43 months after surgery

Conclusions

VSD-I constitutes 34.4% of all the cases of VSD operated in our series. VSD combined with aortic valve lesions is seen in 58.8% of cases of VSD-I and in only 5.6% of cases of VSD-II. There is an increase of surgical cases of VSD-I and associated aortic valve lesions with age. Repair of VSD-I reduced the incidence of AR. After repair of the VSD-I, AR occurred in two older patients, possibly due to the deformed abnormal valve cusp.

No ruptured aneurysm of the sinus of Valsalva was found in repaired VSD-I. The high recurrence rate of AR after valvuloplasty suggests the difficulty of obtaining long-term competency with the deformed abnormal aortic cusp. Early repair of every VSD-I is recommended, particularly when it is combined with aortic valve lesions.

Author Index

Subject Index

Pediatric Cardiology

Proceedings of the Second World Congress
Editors: E. F. Doyle, M. A. Engle, W. M. Gersony, W. J. Rashkind, N. S. Talner

1986. 308 figures. L, 1340 pages. ISBN 3-540-96204-2

Contents: Noninvasive Diagnostic Methods. – Exercise Testing. – Diagnostic and Interventional Cardiac Catheterization. – Cardiac Rhythm Disorders and Electrophysiology. – Cardiovascular Surgery and Surgical Symposia. – Post-Operative Care. – Cardiovascular Nursing. – Cardiac Development; Neonatal Cardiopulmonary Disease and Cardiac Pathology. – Acquired Heart Disorders: Inflammatory Heart Disease and Myocardiopathies. – Heritable Heart Disease; Pediatric Cardiology Practice; and Preventive Cardiology. – Cardiovascular Pharmacology: Symposia on Congestive Heart Failure and Cardiac Glycosides. – Natural History and Long-Term Follow-up.

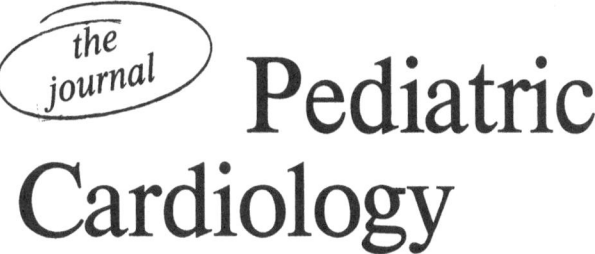

Pediatric Cardiology

Editors: I. Carr, G. Graham (Managing), F. Macartney, R. A. Miller

Springer-Verlag
Tokyo Berlin Heidelberg
New York London Paris

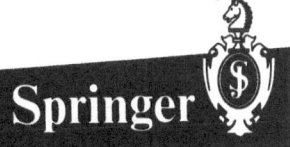

Springer

H. Spindola-Franco, B. G. Fish, New York

Radiology of the Heart

Cardiac Imaging in Infants, Children, and Adults

With contributions by R. Eisenberg, C. B. Higgins, R. M. Steingart, J. P. Wexler

1985. 552 halftone illustrations in 1202 parts plus 62 line illustrations. XVII, 700 pages. ISBN 3-540-90742-4

Radiology of the Heart is a comprehensive, thoroughly illustrated textbook covering all aspects of cardiac radiology in every age group. It describes in full congenital heart malformations, acquired valvular disease, coronary artery disease and cardiomyopathies, and includes modern nuclear and echocardiographic techniques as well as plain films, angiocardiography and coronary arteriography.

Guide to Prosthetic Cardiac Valves

Editors: **D. Morse**, Browns Mills; **R. M. Steiner**, Philadelphia; **J. Fernandez**, Browns Mills

1985. 204 halftone illustrations in 301 parts, 78 line illustrations. XVI, 362 pages. ISBN 3-540-96123-2

This book provides a new approach to various aspects related to the diagnosis and management of patients with valvular heart disease. A wide range of aspects is covered, such as pre- and post-operative care, complications, surgery, pathology, echocardiography, radiologic imaging and bioengineering techniques.

T. Ischinger, Munich

Practice of Coronary Angioplasty

1985. 129 figures, XII, 325 pages. ISBN 3-540-15949-5

This monograph presents different experts' view and practical approaches to percutaneous transluminal coronary angioplasty (PTCA). It informs you of policies of patient selection and patient management, provides detailed description of techniques, describes potential applications, and points out problem areas and limitations of the procedure. Even the experienced angioplasty operator will find useful tips in this state-of-the-art report on PTCA.

Springer-Verlag
Tokyo Berlin Heidelberg
New York London Paris

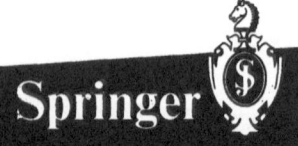

Springer